WRITING
MEDICA~~L PAPERS~~

A prac~~tical~~

CW00969785

Jam~~es Calnan~~

F.R.C.P. (Edin.) M.R.C.P. (Lon~~don~~, ~~B.T.M. and H.,~~
L.D.S., R.C.S., F.C.S.T.

Professor of Plastic and Reconstructive Surgery, (University
of London), Royal Postgraduate Medical School and
Hammersmith Hospital, London.

and

Andras Barabas

M.D., F.R.C.S.

Tutor in Surgery, Royal Postgraduate Medical School and
Hammersmith Hospital London.

WILLIAM HEINEMANN MEDICAL BOOKS LIMITED

First Published 1973

Illustrations mainly by Andras Barabas. Cover design by Cherry Calnan

© 1973 J. Calnan and A. Barabas

ISBN 0 433 05005 5

Text set in 9/10 pt. Monotype Times New Roman, printed by
photolithography, and bound in Great Britain at The Pitman Press, Bath

FOREWORD

There is an ancient Chinese proverb which says that anyone who can write his name can draw. Like all such proverbs it contains a truth and no doubt, with much hard work and application, there are few who could not make some showing in the field of art. The same is true of writing and doctors spend a deal of time, pen in hand. What they need however is someone to help them express themselves clearly and this is just what Professor Calnan and Mr Barabas have done.

The amount of wisdom which the senior author has distilled into this little book is out of all proportion to its size. His style is lucid, attractive yet artlessly unadorned. It is most reminiscent of that master medical writer Richard Asher and, like him, the authors poke fun at all pretentiousness and circumlocution. The text is admirably illustrated by Barabas' drawings which have the pungent wit of the cartoonist.

I have made a New Year resolution to present a copy of this little book to each assistant who comes to work with me. It is the best guide I know to preparing a medical paper and if it is true that the young doctor must publish or be damned, salvation was never had so cheaply.

I commend this book to all aspiring medical authors.

SELWYN TAYLOR

Royal Postgraduate Medical School,
Hammersmith Hospital,
London, W12 OHS.

TABLE OF CONTENTS

INTRODUCTION

Much has been done to improve medical writing. Editors reject ill-prepared scripts and attempt to improve those accepted. Adjudicators and referees provide detailed criticism of the content of papers submitted so that a journal may retain its high standards in the face of the volume of work presented to it.

Yet many authors find difficulty in placing a piece of writing which has taken much time and trouble to prepare and may contain work of importance. Writing, like every other practical art, cannot be learned wholly from books or in the class-room. Books such as the present can survey the field, can point the way the beginner should follow, can even smooth over some of the difficulties. But the art, the craft, can be learned only 'on the job'. The best teachers have always been, and always will be, the beginner's own more experienced colleagues.

The staff of the Royal Postgraduate Medical School and Hammersmith Hospital produce over 600 publications in reputable journals all over the world every year. The majority are well written and advance knowledge. Why is it that one institution can provide an output equal to three other hospitals in the same city? We believe that the answer lies as much in the training and expertise of writing as it does in the quality of the material proffered; it is not so much the value of the work but the manner of presenting it.

Good medical writing is creative, and we believe well within the capability of every medically qualified person. Naturally, it should be informative, but the act of writing can be pleasurable too. There are already many books published on the subject, and our only excuse for another is that we have tried to produce a practical manual which we hope will complement our earlier 'Speaking at Medical Meetings'.

A. THE AUTHORS

1

THE JUNIOR DOCTOR

'It is terrible to have no means of expressing oneself, always to have
to keep one's feelings a secret.'

Somerset Maugham

The Junior Doctor, whether he intends to join the ranks of medical
authors or not, cannot escape a certain amount of writing. He has to
write answers to examination questions to become qualified in his
profession, and later he has to apply often for a series of appointments. Later still, he may be angry at what he has read and so write
to the editor of a journal, and finally, he may see a clinical condition
which to him appears to be so unusual that he is driven to publish it.

1. Writing an Examination Paper

In medicine, more than any other profession, multiple examinations
have to be endured and passed. Training at medical school for
qualification and later for a higher degree may mean that a man has
to spend ten years studying, with the sole object of sitting and passing
these written examinations (Fig. 1).

Some people know enough about the subject but are unable to
organize their thoughts and so write clearly within the time available.
Others can write fluently but often do not answer the question asked,
from lack of correct interpretation. It helps to remember that a
discipline in this as in other writing, can be developed with a little
practice and that there are 4 points to consider:

1. Read the question slowly and underline the key words. There
is a wealth of difference between 'Discuss the difficulties in diagnosis
of . . .', and, 'discuss the diagnosis of . . .'.

2. Think about the question and jot down notes as the answer
begins to form in your own mind. Five to seven minutes spent in this
way is well repaid.

3. Rearrange the ideas in a sequential and logical order, for clarity and the avoidance of repetition.

4. Then begin to write legibly and start a new paragraph for each new idea you wish to record. Remember that there is a time limit and so if there are 3 questions to be answered within 2 hours, the actual

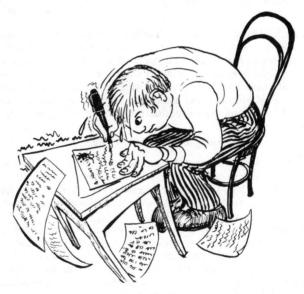

Fig. 1.

writing time for each question will be little more than 30 minutes. The final act is to read over what has been written, for punctuation and correct spelling; revision, except in a very limited way, is never practicable.

4

2. Applying for a Post

For the junior doctor this is the commonest chore in writing and the easiest to do badly. Most institutions have a form of application to complete and this should always be requested unless the advertisement of the post clearly states otherwise.

In applying for a post, the object is to sell your abilities by presenting yourself in the best light (Fig. 2). Initially you will be a paper

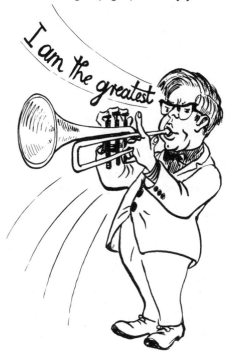

Fig. 2.

applicant, so it is wise to read the advertisement several times to make sure that you are applying for the appropriate job.

All your qualifications should be recorded. If you have attended courses for instance, in computers, teaching, or audio-visual aids, and have become expert in these areas this should be stated along with your purely medical experience.

A suggested format would be as follows:

1. Name, address, age (date of birth in brackets), marital state, number of children, nationality.
2. Education: name of school, University, and of hospital where trained.
3. Qualifications with dates.
4. Academic distinctions.
5. Present appointment.
6. Previous appointments and grading: give details.
7. Detail of any further experience.
8. Membership of societies.
9. Publications: give journal references and titles.
10. Research projects undertaken.
11. Names of referees to whom application may be made for references.
12. Any additional information. Particular interests, intended career.
13. Signature of the candidate and the date.

The covering letter can be quite brief but the application itself should be typed because it is more than likely to be photocopied for perusal by members of the selection committee. If the names of two referees are requested, do not give three, and remember always to write to them asking permission for this favour well in advance; few people object to supporting a candidate but most feel annoyed at having to compose a eulogy at short notice and without prior warning (*and see* Asher 1972, p. 124).

6

It is useless to enclose testimonials which cannot have any real value for the selection committee. If they were not praiseworthy you would not even consider them in the first place, and everyone realises this; they are bound to be incomplete and may not even be truthful.

All spaces in the application should be completed even if one has to write 'Nil' for previous publications; in this section a list of papers in preparation does not impress. If confirmation of receipt of the application is required, enclosing a stamped and addressed post-card will be appreciated by the administration; if you wish to know if you have not been short-listed for the job, enclose another with an appropriate message.

It is of course, wise to be well-dressed at the interview, and you should be quite clear what you expect from the post, and what it entails; if there has been any doubt, a prior visit to survey the scene is rarely out of order. Some applicants think that mentioning an interest in research will help their appointment, but have no specific problem or ideas to discuss when asked; yet a little thought beforehand could have prevented an embarrassing situation. If you have no idea of how to go about it, then it is better not to bring up the subject at all. It is important to be natural, and not to look unfriendly, suspicious or aggressive; to be obsequious is worst of all. A set speech is a mistake because it will clearly lack spontaneity and may leave the impression that you have become a professional 'job-seeker'.

3. A Case Report

We have noticed that the medical student who writes articles for his hospital journal or gazette, often goes on to contribute to the general scientific medical literature. He has appreciated the art of writing well and enjoyed it. Clearly such writing is good practice for later life.

Many a young doctor has felt that he must publish a scientific paper or two to further his career, yet does not know how to go about it. He may recognize a problem, or have collected a significant amount of material but cannot set it down. It is usually easier to start by writing a case report of an unusual finding or of a rare disease. All that appears necessary is to type out the history, the clinical findings, the special investigations and the results of treatment, in exactly the same order as they were recorded in the patient's notes, to add a few illustrations to the script and then submit it to an appropriate journal. The section on 'discussion' may require a little more effort for the author has to ask himself why the patient had symptoms, why things happened as they did, and why the therapeutic result turned out the way it did. Surprisingly, the paper may be accepted and published and he congratulates himself on his expertise. Unfortunately, his next paper is less successful; he then feels hurt and frustrated.

There are few opportunities for witty writing in medicine. The case report is one of them. Yet such reports are generally dull reading. The facts are recorded, the literature inadequately searched, but the opportunity for pungent descriptive writing is lost. Asher's papers (1972), now published as a book, the work of Roueche (1966), are examples of interesting reporting and powerful writing.

Although a structure for writing is desirable in the sequence of history, examination, investigation, treatment, and subsequent outcome, there is no need to follow this rigidly. The 'introduction' should be brief, and any references held for the 'discussion', which may occupy half the report. Editors welcome reports on unusual cases because they so frequently help to fill the empty 1–2 pages found when making up the next issue of the journal. For that reason alone, publication is often speedy. This should not, however, lead the author to think that he can put his gem together quickly. The same care as in writing a longer paper is demanded, and the same amount of rewriting and revision will be required.

4. A Letter to a Journal

Some medical journals have correspondence columns and in our opinion there are too few of them. We know of doctors whose only literary effort has been a letter to the Lancet, and even that was badly done. In writing a letter, thought and time are required. The reasons for writing are commonly:

1. To comment on an article which has appeared recently in the same journal. Whether expressing agreement or disagreement the writer should provide supporting evidence for his views and avoid libellous statements.

2. To broach a subject which cannot be raised in any other way. Editors welcome controversial correspondence because it stimulates others to join in and may provoke lively writing.

3. To publish preliminary work of importance which may not yet warrant a full length article. In this way priority can be achieved in the field, but the complete paper should follow within a reasonable time. Letters to 'Nature' are of this kind, and most journals will print simple line drawings as easily as text.

The three common faults to avoid are: pompous circumlocution about trivia, self-opinionated statements, and the lack of factual information. All three can be heard at the club bar, but should not appear in print.

Every letter requires a structure:

1. Start with the greeting—'Sir'—since all letters are addressed to the editor of the journal. There is no need therefore, to send a covering letter unless you feel strongly that your personal reasons for writing should be made known but not published.

2. The introduction, of one sentence, should explain why you are writing. If it refers to a paper published earlier, the reference should be given at the end. One or two references necessary to support your own arguments should also be recorded in full.

3. The main message should be a simple statement which can then be developed sufficiently for the purpose, either to convince others or to contradict. Simplicity is the most sought-after quality in art and nature, so why not in writing?

4. State your conclusions briefly: to put it more bluntly—sum up and stop.

5. Finish by signing your name and giving your address. Editors do not like printing anonymous letters, but will do so if the author in a covering letter provides serious reasons for not wishing his name to be known.

It is important to have something worth-while to say. If you do not, then by all means write a letter, but don't post it (Fig. 3).

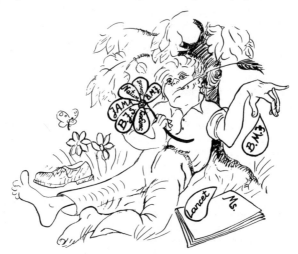

Fig. 3.

5. Which Journal?

The most suitable journal for your publication will depend on several factors:

1. The general quality of your paper and the prestige of the journal in which you wish to publish.

2. The size and circulation of the journal. What public do you desire to reach? Will the paper be of interest generally or is it intended for the specialist? Does the journal have editorial and correspondence sections? Will these be important to you?

3. Speed of publication: is this important? How long is the waiting list for the journal in which you would like to place it? Several journals print the date of submission as a footnote to each paper and from looking at several it is easy to calculate the average waiting time; with weekly journals it is usually short, but in specialist journals it may be over one year.

4. Your illustrations may require good quality paper for accurate reproduction which will necessarily limit the choice.

5. Examine the journal for the type of material selected. Fashions change and some journals are pleased to expand their range of subjects to attract a larger reading public.

6. Read the editorial notices, note the editorial committee and directions about submission. Familiarity with the lay-out of papers, how the references are set out and how long the summary should be are clearly important. Is the summary at the beginning or at the end of papers?

You will have to ask some fairly searching questions, such as whether the work is original in your own country, and whether it is sufficiently important for the journal of choice. When it has been written, it is advisable to consider the choice of journal again, as well as the soundness of the statistics, the logic and the quality of writing.

6. Sending it to the Editor

When the paper has been typed and any errors in the top copy corrected in black ink, it should be sent to the editor of one journal only with a short covering note. If the work is entirely new or raises serious doubts about a paper published earlier in the same journal, it is worth saying so. Most general medical journals submit papers to referees before acceptance; hence it is often worth enclosing a second copy of the script and tables, with photocopies of any figures, so that the editor can send your paper to two referees at once, and so save time. Always keep a copy for your own files.

Usually within 6–8 weeks, the editor will reply. His letter may indicate one of three decisions:

1. Outright acceptance, but this is uncommon.

2. A request for revision of the script, usually to shorten it but sometimes to amplify a particular passage. If only minor revisions are required these should be carried through quickly, the relevant pages retyped, and the whole returned. The accompanying letter should state what has been changed, and thank the referee for his comments.

If major alterations are required, then you have to ask yourself, 'Is it worth it?' If you decide to go ahead it is usually better to have the whole paper retyped. When re-submitting the paper the original manuscript should be enclosed so that the editor can see that you have followed his advice. If you decide not to resubmit, then proceed as below.

3. Out-right rejection. The editor may state that the paper is too specialized for his journal (often the truth), that it is unsuitable (meaning that it is not very good), or that he has no space (which often means that it's pretty bad). You can do one of four things:

i. Amend the manuscript and send it to another journal, but only if the editor has said 'too specialized'.
ii. Consider modifying the length and content of the whole article, having noted the criticisms offered by referees, and submitting it to another journal.
iii. Withhold the paper until you have more data. This is often the wisest choice, but the most difficult to make.
iv. Contest the editor's decision, which we do not advise (Fig. 4).

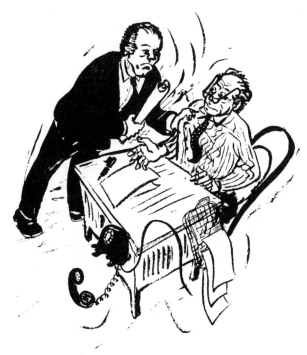

Fig. 4.

7. Proofs

In due course you will receive proofs of your paper. You should read through these carefully for:

i. accuracy of spelling;

ii. any omissions, which is unusual, but such may alter the sense of what you have written;

iii. comprehension. Reading the proofs is not an opportunity for rewriting your paper. If however, you now find that he meaning in one of your sentences is obscure, you should correct it but keep alterations to a minimum; often the substitution of a single word is all that is necessary. Alterations are expensive, so try to keep the same number of characters in the new text as in the printed line.

There are special notations used in printing for corrections which are shown below and see Trelease, 1955: it is not absolutely necessary to know these but you should record all corrections in the covering letter to the editor, written within 3 days of reception, when returning proofs. At the same time, order the number of reprints you think you may require.

Printers Corrections

The list of symbols shown ('B.S. 1219c: 1958 Table of symbols for printers' and authors' proof corrections') is reproduced by permission of the British Standards Institution, 2 Park Street, London, W1A 2BS, from whom copies of the complete standard may be obtained.

SYMBOLS FOR CORRECTING PROOFS

No.	Instruction	Textual mark	Marginal mark
1	Correction is concluded	None	/
2	Insert in text the matter indicated in margin	⋀	*New matter followed by* /
3	Delete	Strike through characters to be deleted	ℐ
4	Delete and close up	Strike through characters to be deleted and use mark 21	ℐ

No.	Instruction	Textual mark	Marginal mark
5	Leave as printed	. . . . under characters to remain	*stet*
6	Change to italic	_____ under characters to be altered	*ital*
7	Change to even small capitals	═══ under characters to be altered	*s.c.*
8	Change to capital letters	≡≡≡ under characters to be altered	*caps*
9	Use capital letters for initial letters and small capitals for rest of words	≡≡≡ under initial letters and ═══ under the rest of the words	*c. & s.c.*
10	Change to bold type	⌇⌇⌇ under characters to be altered	*bold*
11	Change to lower case	Encircle characters to be altered	*l.c.*
12	Change to roman type	Encircle characters to be altered	*rom*
13	Change damaged character(s)	Encircle character(s) to be altered	X
14	Substitute or insert character(s) under which this mark is placed, in 'superior' position	/ through character or ⋏ where required	⋎ *under character* (e.g. ⋎)
15	Substitute or insert character(s) over which this mark is placed, in 'inferior' position	/ through character or ⋏ where required	⋀ *over character* (e.g. ⋀)
16	Underline word or words	_____ under words affected	‾‾ *underline*
17	Close up—delete space between characters	⌒ linking characters	⌣
18	Insert space*	⋏	#

15

No.	Instruction	Textual mark	Marginal mark
19	Insert space between lines or paragraphs*	`>` between lines to be spaced	#
20	Reduce space between lines*	`(` connecting lines to be closed up	less #
21	Make space appear equal between words	`|` between words	eq #
22	Reduce space between words*	`|` between words	less #
23	Add space between letters*	`ιιιιι` between tops of letters requiring space	letter #
24	Transpose	`⌐⌐` between characters or words, numbered when necessary	trs
25	Move matter to right	`⌐` at left side of group to be moved	⌐
26	Move matter to left	`⌐` at right side of group to be moved	⌐
27	Move matter to position indicated	`[    ]` at limits of required position	move
28	Begin a new paragraph	`[` before first word of new paragraph	n.p.
29	No fresh paragraph here	`⌐` between paragraphs	run on
30	Spell out the abbreviation or figure in full	Encircle words or figures to be altered	spell out
31	Insert omitted portion of copy NOTE. The relevant section of the copy should be returned with the proof, the omitted portion being clearly indicated.	`λ`	out see copy
32	Substitute or insert comma	`/` through character or `λ` where required	,/

16

No.	Instruction	Textual mark	Marginal mark
33	Substitute or insert semi-colon	/ through character or ⋏ where required	;/
34	Substitute or insert full stop	/ through character or ⋏ where required	⊙
35	Substitute or insert colon	/ through character or ⋏ where required	⊙
36	Substitute or insert interrogation mark	/ through character or ⋏ where required	?/
37	Substitute or insert exclamation mark	/ through character or ⋏ where required	!/
38	Insert parentheses	⋏ or ⋏ ⋏	(/)/
39	Insert (square) brackets	⋏ or ⋏ ⋏	[/]/
40	Insert hyphen	⋏	|-|
41	Insert apostrophe	⋏	⸍
42	Insert single quotation marks	⋏ or ⋏ ⋏	⸍ ⸍
43	Insert double quotation marks	⋏ or ⋏ ⋏	⸌⸍ ⸌⸍

8. Readability

Every newspaper editor is acutely aware of this subject: the more readable his paper, the larger the circulation. Yet, by and large, most medical authors never give it a second thought.

Gunning (1968), in his book has produced a formula for budding authors by which to judge readability. The number of words in a passage, say a page of manuscript, is divided by the number of sentences. Then the number of three or more syllable words is counted in every 100 words, which gives the percentage of hard words in a passage. The sum of these two factors multiplied by 0·4 is the 'fog index' (Fig. 5). Gunning believed, from his own research,

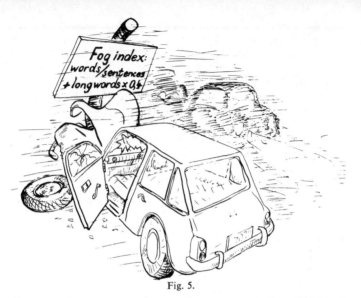

Fig. 5.

that an index of 12 was the danger point: scores higher then this indicated that a script was becoming difficult to read. He also stated that sentences which averaged more than 20 words made difficult reading. We have summarized in one page all that Gunning wrote in his 300! His book is well-worth reading for he also provides ten principles of clear writing, with examples which should be noted.

Not everyone would agree that Medicine, with its vast number of polysyllable technical terms, can be subjected to the same treatment. This may be so. All we are saying is that Gunning provides a standard or ideal towards which we should all try to work; as he so rightly says, the 'fog index' should be used as a guide after you have written, not as a pattern before. Good writing must be alive, not stodgy, but a literary style with an average complexity within the 6–12 range is likely to be better understood.

Hence, it is wise to keep sentences short, but the great secret is variety. Good writers tend not to have more than two or three subordinate clauses in one sentence; if there should be more, the wise man will divide his script into two sentences of unequal length, or abolish the qualifying phrases which are not really necessary. The common fault with the beginner is trying to say too much in one sentence. Lawyers, too, have the odd notion that it is better to cram all ideas into one sentence, and so it is little wonder that legal documents make such difficult reading.

The readability of writing depends largely on:

1. its dramatic effect which holds the reader;
2. the easy flowing style;
3. the perfection of composition and grammar;
4. its clarity and completeness.

9. Style

A lot has been written about style (Quiller-Couch, 1916, Strunk and White, 1959). Style is the way that you and I write. Good style implies the use of language which conveys the writer's meaning clearly, is grammatically accurate, and is appropriate to the subject matter. A sentence should be smooth, but if it is ambiguous then something clumsier and unequivocal is better; the cardinal sin is vagueness, not bad grammar. Brevity is an advantage, but a long precise statement is better than a short obscure one. A distinctive style is a personal characteristic which can be acquired by reading good literature, and certainly not by imitating current scientific writing. Elegant writing demands selective reading.

Style is also to do with your relationship to your reader. It is neither a garnish added afterwards, nor an ornament to dress it up for greater impressiveness. Style depends on:

1. Confidence in writing, which improves with practice.
2. Authority, that is, knowing the subject well.

3. Rhythm of writing; well written means well thought out, so be sensitive to the cadence of the language.

There are some general rules which help to develop an individual and interesting style:

1. Be simple and concise in important statements.
2. Make sure of the meaning of every word. The more clearly you write, the more easily and surely you will be understood.
3. Use verbs instead of abstract nouns.
4. Break up noun clusters and modifiers; it is usually advisable to allow only two together. Baker (1955) condemned the German-American style of using multiple noun qualifiers, especially those long words derived from Latin and Greek roots, when a simple word will do. This is called grandiloquence, and allied to it is genteelism ('sacrificed' for 'killed'). The use of archaic words ('save' for 'except') and vogue words shows that you are not merely illiterate, but pretentious.
5. Use analogies to explain difficult or unfamiliar matters and thus produce a sense of intimacy with your reader. These are introduced by 'as' and 'like'; they have visual appeal which helps us to see and remember. Analogy is a most useful way of introducing and developing a subject, but does not constitute logical proof. However, a good analogy reveals more than a general resemblance for its details must be meaningful.
6. Metaphors help to provide a word picture, but one should try to make up new comparisons and abandon the common clichés. Metaphors and similes are richly suggestive for they can expand the writer's meaning in a few words.
7. The use of summarizing phrases, 'in other words', 'in short', 'in brief', allow the reader to digest your writing more easily.
8. The insertion of questions varies the pace of reading.
9. Repetition when required should be made in different words, but remember that repetition is essentially for the spoken lecture and not for the written paper.
10. Use expressive, distinctive words in short sentences.

11. Ask what can be shortened? What can be simplified? What can be eliminated altogether? Verbose writing is commonly inaccurate.

12. Finally, look at word order. The normal order is subject, verb, object but this is often the least emphatic. Altering the order may produce a different impact.

Style is largely a matter of taste and of the character of the journal in which your paper is published, of the decade, of the author, and perhaps too of clarity. The main essentials are the writer, the reader, and the material. It is therefore advisable to adapt your style to the readership, to make your prose various and interesting. Good style is recognized by the reader as easy reading.

It is important for every author of scientific writing to lay the firm foundation of his own style in the first publication. Improvement will come with experience, but the ideal should be aimed for at the start. Perhaps the most useful style for scientific writing is tightly knit factual prose, but we have more to say about that in a later section.

10. In Defence of Writing

Writing is most beneficial for the author, not the reader. It is good mental discipline to collect data, organize it and then reduce it to a lucid written form. As Bacon noted, 'writing maketh an exact man'. Writing may determine your own professional immortality (Fig. 6), hence, great care in accuracy and logic should be expended in preparing a permanent record for all to consult, which cannot be forgotten like speech. In spite of that, most of us fail to view our own writing critically and objectively, so that the literature has become cluttered with valueless material, as many of your colleagues will be quick to point out. We maintain that this is not a good reason to avoid putting pen to paper, but a very good reason for taking care in what you write.

It helps to remember that there are three types of writing in medicine:

(a) Narration, tells a story and the material is arranged in a time sequence. A case report of an unusual disease can be set out

21

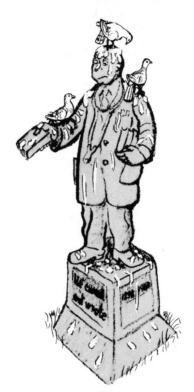

Fig. 6.

in this way and every medical student is taught to record the case history of his patients thus.

(b) Description, or how something looks. The theme is organized in space and an example would be the description of a new piece of apparatus.

22

(c) Exposition, which explains the how, what and why in most scientific writing, and is organized by logic. This is the commonest form of writing in medical journals and we shall deal with this in detail.

In defence of writing we would state that there is much to be gained for the individual.

1. Even boring subjects become interesting if you take the trouble to sort them out and are sufficiently curious to try to make them interesting.

2. The effort of placing one word in front of another with economy and lucidity is a lost art for most doctors, but an invaluable discipline.

3. Writing adds a new dimension to the understanding of any clinical condition.

4. Scholarship is the intellectual counterpart of manual dexterity in clinical work, and is therefore just as necessary for every professional man who is not prepared to decline into a pure technician.

5. Writing helps to establish the personality of every doctor as an individual. It is good for his ego and may be good for the other labourers in medicine if he has something new to say. There is also the fun of writing, and a little 'gamesmanship' in addition.

Whether one writes for publication or not, and of course most of us do, there are 6 good reasons why work should be published:

1. To report the unusual or unexpected in medicine so that others may be warned. Such are case reports and brief notes on the ill effect of drugs.

2. To report experimental research which may or may not have immediate clinical applications, or the results of clinical research which may affect current practice. The results of a controlled clinical trial in therapy is an example of the latter.

3. To report a new condition, a new treatment, or the analysis of a series of patients with a rare condition, and so add to the general body of medical knowledge.

4. To describe new inventions, equipment, instruments, or improved diagnostic and therapeutic agents.

5. To review current practice and the results of treatment at one institute so that others may compare. Review articles chapters in text books and retrospective studies are of this nature.

6. To propose an hypothesis based on observations; but remember that some proof of its validity will be required from the author. Sadly for most of us, nearly all our bright ideas fall short when put to the test. 'The tragedy of science is the slaying of beautiful ideas by ugly facts' (T. H. Huxley).

2

THE MORE SENIOR DOCTOR

'If politics is the art of the possible, research is surely the art of the soluble. Both are immensely practical-minded affairs'

Sir Peter Medawar

The more senior doctor in training will of necessity have to write reports, if only about patients at the request of those who control the finances of a state health service. He may also be delegated by his chief to investigate a clinical condition, and perhaps report on it at a scientific meeting. Writing is coming to be a way of life.

1. Writing Reports

Many doctors do not enjoy writing reports; they consider them time-wasting procedures when there is so much practical work to be done in treating patients and in the research laboratory. This is a mistaken view. A well written factual report may become a valuable document for the author and the receiver. As Cooper (1964) points out, it is the crucial test of a person's knowledge to be explicit and articulate, to make it intelligible to others. 'This is surely the difference between the technologist and the technician.' The fact that a doctor looks upon report writing as the least important and necessary of his activities, is no excuse for doing it badly.

The writing of a report differs from the writing of a paper for publication in three important aspects—the specificity of its content, the known readership, and the limited time for preparation. Reports are demanded and so those who ask have to read them. You, therefore, have captive readers. If writing a report is an unwelcome chore, reading it is often an unnecessary bore. Great literary style is not expected, but brevity and clarity are appreciated. Even if the readership is known in advance, the interest will not be uniformly shared. Those who will be most affected by your report will read in detail and probably talk it over with you later; those least affected will scan it quickly and if it is difficult to understand, will file it away without being any the wiser. Before putting pen to paper ask yourself: Who is it for? What is it about? How long should it be?

There are two general principles which apply to the writing of all reports. These concern the structure and the layout.

A. Structure of a Report

A report conveys specific information to a specific reader and requires a structure like any other piece of writing. Because time for its preparation may be limited, the first draft may have to be the final composition. It his therefore doubly important to write concisely and clearly and to use simple familiar words in uncomplicated sentences. If you think that your report will require about 6000 words, try to reduce it to 3000 and put the supporting information that is really necessary in an 'appendix'.

The plan of a report should be as follows:

1. The title page, with your name, the date of the report, and for whom it is intended (its circulation).
2. If the report is more than 5000 words a contents page is a good idea.
3. The next page should be an abstract if the report is longer than 5 typed pages. This should contain all the essential facts and be so constructed that it can be circulated alone to other interested parties as the article in miniature.
4. The introduction should tell the reader why the investigation was made, how it was carried out, and what were the chief findings. You do not have to capture the reader's attention as for a published paper, but you have to hold it. The introduction should therefore be simple, short, and direct.
5. The main body of the report requires an orderly presentation. A chronological sequence is ideal for a medical report on a patient but unsuitable for a research report, even though the work was done in a chronological order. It is important to decide on the most

appropriate format and to arrange the observations within it before constructing the prose. One should deal with simple facts and ideas before recording the more complex, so that the reader is led logically on.

6. Interpretation may not be called for if the facts speak for themselves. If they do not, then an hypothesis to explain them is required; since this is often a personal interpretation, the use of 'I' or 'we' is in order. There is a curious notion that objectivity can only be obtained by writing impersonally. We entirely disagree and would argue strongly for personal involvement of the writer in any report. We also disagree with the notion that vagueness is in some way the same as being diplomatic.

7. The main recommendations constitute the most important part of the report for the busy reader. If the main facts and arguments have been well set out, he has a simple decision to make, either to agree or disagree. If there are no recommendations then this section should contain the conclusions, cogently expressed.

8. References, if any.

9. Appendices, if required. These should contain extra detail for the selective and interested reader, which do not form an essential part of the main report.

B. The Lay-Out

Lay-out is important: it should not be left to the secretary who types or stencils your report. An attractive appearance to a report tells the reader immediately that you have taken trouble. Furthermore, a durable cover allows your work to be handled frequently, and passed to others without looking unkempt. The cover should be transparent, to allow the title to be seen, or if opaque, of a distinctive colour with the title boldly set out. A faceless report quickly becomes lost on anyone's desk. We believe that the following are important for good appearance and ease of reading.

1. Each new section should start on a new page.
2. Sub-headings should be used frequently so that the reader can

consume a small quantity and perhaps a new idea, piecemeal. He will also follow the structure of the report more easily.

3. Paragraphs should be used discreetly to break up the typed page. A sheet of solid type is hardly conducive to detailed reading.

4. Tables should be inserted so that they can be seen at the right time within the script. If there are about 250 words to a page of type, it is not difficult to insure that tables are inserted in the correct place.

5. Diagrams and graphs, drawn in black ink, should be used and be continuous with the script if they facilitate the reader's understanding of your message and allow the script to be shorter. If the report is to be duplicated, it is usually easier to have the illustrations photocopied rather than draw them on a stencil sheet. Alternatively, they can be photocopied, trimmed and mounted on the typed sheet.

6. If you produce an artistic and neat work, your appreciative reader is more likely to look it over again and so better understand what you have written.

2. A Medical Report (for Litigation)

One morning a letter arrives on your desk from a solicitor asking for a medical report on a patient whom you have seen at some time. You may not remember the patient and the letter rarely indicates the reason for the requests; usually there is no signature of an individual, only the anonymous 'X and Co.' What are you to do?

Naturally you will look up the patient's records. If she has not been seen for some months you will wish to send her an appointment so that the examination will be up to date. The solicitor's letter should be acknowledged, the date you intend to see his client included and a specific enquiry made whether the patient has agreed to the disclosure of confidential information to him. At this stage it is in order to mention your fee for the medical report.

The medical report should be set out under 4 headings:

1. History.
2. Examination.

3. Further treatment required, if any.
4. Assessment.

1. History

Naturally, this will include all the relevant information of events and symptoms, provided by the patient as in normal clinical practice. Most of the information will be found in the patient's records but since you will have seen the patient again any important features not recorded earlier should be included, with a remark that such were discovered on later questioning.

This section should include all events which preceded the most recent examination, including treatment, special investigations and the results, length of stay in hospital, dates of subsequent review, when the patient returned to work and how she fared. Everything should be recorded in chronological order.

2. Examination

The date of the examination should be mentioned, and this section includes the patient's symptoms as well as the clinical findings at the time. If special investigations were made, the result of these should be noted. The idea is to present to the solicitor a picture of the patient at one moment in time. Hence, if the patient suffered injuries from a road-traffic accident (and it is foolish not to record details when the patient is first seen, because so many become litigenous) measurement of the length of scars with a note of their condition and site (including a diagram if thought necessary) must be stated quite clearly.

3. Further Treatment

If it is considered advisable, or likely, that further treatment will be required to obtain the best result, this must be stated: a note of fees, stay in hospital and time off work should be included, whether the patient avails herself of this advice or not.

4. Assessment

Assessment should take account of three aspects and the importance of each mentioned:

(a) Disfigurement
(b) Deformity
(c) Disability.

Assessment is the most difficult part of the report to write well because it depends largely on opinion and on previous personal experience. One of us uses the following preamble: 'I always find assessment difficult. It is not my practice to assess deformity, disability or disfigurement on a percentage basis, but rather to use the terms slight, moderate or severe. For instance, to most people the loss of the little finger of the left hand would be considered slight, but to a concert violinist the disability would be severe. In the case of Mrs X I assess the deformity as . . . the disability as . . ., etc.'

It is also important in most instances to state whether the disability, deformity or disfigurement will improve spontaneously with time. Assessment of the severity of headaches, insomnia and other unmeasurable symptoms is much more difficult, and can usually be covered by a general sentence recording the patient's complaint in her own words.

The whole report should be written in clear, concise English, and in the usual medical terms. Abbreviations should not be used, unless a particular group of words is repeated frequently. It is essential, of course, in writing the assessment to know exactly the patient's occupation; if it is unfamiliar, you should obtain details so that you can categorize the job as skilled or unskilled.

3. Applying for Research Funds

Rightly or wrongly, a great many junior doctors believe that they have to do research in order to obtain an interesting senior appointment. (There will always be some expert around to advise you otherwise, that your job is to treat patients, not to live in a lab.) We do not intend to argue either way but would point out that research has an educational function for education is the accumulation of experience, not facts. (Welbourn, 1966.) Sooner or later, it will be necessary to apply for finances to support the research project. It is never too soon to apply, for it may take 3–6 months to succeed. How is one to go about it? (Fig. 7).

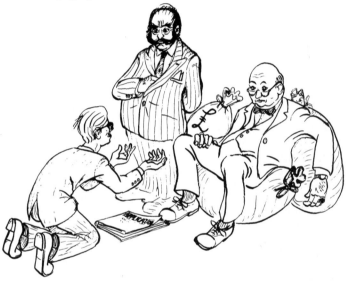

Fig. 7.

Doris Merritt (1963) has described the application for funds as 'grantmanship: an exercise in lucid presentation', and Allen (1960) has recorded some of the reasons why grants are not approved, and these are usually self-inflicted wounds. We suggest that an application for funds, like an application for anything else, should have a certain

31

structure and provide information clearly and concisely. Writing the application will require as much thought, and nearly as much time as a paper for publication. We propose the following format, with each heading starting on a new page unless the donors, such as the Medical Research Council, have their own form to be completed.

1. A title page which should carry a short descriptive title, the applicant's name and address, and the date of submission.

2. The introduction should provide a very brief summary of the problem it is proposed to tackle, and only a few relevant references to previous work need be given. A good method is to pose questions which are of importance and which you seek to answer. These can, and perhaps should, be provocative. They are likely to interest the reader and persuade him that the application is important.

3. Methods and materials (or plan of the investigation) The description of both should be explicit. It requires considerable judgement to know how much to include, but the application should contain sufficient detail to allow another to carry out the work as planned. If analytical methods are well known then a single reference to a published paper is all that is required. If, however, new methods are introduced they should be defined in detail; if they are long and complex it may be more convenient to place them at the end, as an appendix. One has to explain complexities in terms which will be recognized by the reader and in words which permit of only one interpretation. You have to demonstrate by irrefutable logic and imaginative insight that there is a gap in knowledge to be filled.

If it is likely that one method may succeed and another fail, then alternative methods should be included. The successful applications are those which contain a well-defined problem and a well-defined approach. If pilot studies have been carried out, showing that the work is feasible, they should be recorded with all the preliminary data.

4. Facilities available. These should be described accurately. If certain equipment is required it should be intimated, and its cost included in the budget. It is also advisable to mention the names of experts who are available for consultation or technical help.

5. Where the work will be done should always be specified. If certain measurements are to be made at another institute this must be stated and the consent of any collaborator mentioned.

6. The curriculum vitae of the chief investigator can be included here, or as an appendix, and will also include pertinent previous publications. This section is important, for by it the assessor may be able to judge the background of the applicant and his potential ability in research.

7. Finances required. These should be set out as:

    (a) Capital costs

    (b) Recurrent expenses.

It is realistic to ask for what is required to complete the job. One should ask for money to cover the time that will be devoted to the research. In the U.K. a three-year limit is commonly enforced, so if the research is likely to take 5 years it may be worth dividing it into two projects, the second to be supported when the first is finished. The cost of personnel (salary, superannuation, increments), animals and their husbandry, materials and other disposable items should be accurate.

8. References must be relevant and recent. You should have read them and judged their importance and applicability. If they do not support your proposed work, do not include them.

All applications to grant-giving bodies are referred to a consultant, or other expert in the field for his advice. He will examine your application and ask 5 questions, the answers to which should be obvious from your writing.

1. Is it important?
2. Can it be done?
3. Is the investigator competent to carry out the work?
4. Can it be done within the specified time?
5. Are the costs realistic?

Applications are turned down commonly because:

1. They have little scientific merit.
2. The work is based on an unsound hypothesis, is more complex

than the investigator realized, is premature, or the description is too nebulous, diffuse, and obscure. The error here is in not taking sufficient trouble and time to think about the project, or just plain ignorance.

3. Lack of design, inadequate methods and inexperience with the techniques proposed.

4. Excessive reliance on others to carry out the major part of the work, and general lack of common sense on the part of the investigator.

4. Reporting Research

Most grant-giving bodies expect a report at the end of the year on what you have done with their money. This need not be long but should be factual and to the point. If your grant is for three years you may not have a great deal to say in the first year's report. If the work is going well, say so; if it is going badly, explain the difficulties. The report should always be typed.

A basic structure will be required as in writing any report:

1. The first page should define the title of the research, include the names of all those taking part, it should record whether it is the first, second, or third report, and indicate the date of submission.

2. The introduction should explain what work the grant was given for, if this is not clear from the title.

3. Progress of the work will form the major portion and this can be recorded chronologically. Details of material and methods are not required, but tentative conclusions should be included. If an important discovery has been made then it is your duty to inform the grants committee, for they too may have to raise money by public subscription and any such information helps their task.

If part of the work has been presented to a learned society this should be recorded, with the date.

4. If you have published a paper on the subject, a reprint should be enclosed: some ask for two. The investigator often forgets this duty, but it is likely to influence the grant-giving body in providing further support.

5. Publishing Research

Many doctors carry out a piece of research moderately successfully and then find difficulty in writing well or even having it published. This is doing things the wrong way round. Others have no idea how to start.

There are many reasons for wanting to do research: for curiosity, prestige, idealism or the imitation of others. Successful research requires average intelligence, simple curiosity, intense preoccupation, ambition and motivation. A sense of showmanship and selfishness are valuable assets. The value of research to the individual lies in the wider horizon of science provided, the concentration of thought required, the reading in depth of the subject necessary, and the self-discipline demanded. The gift of the laboratory lies in its discipline in scientific method, its training in the importance of logical reasoning, and the use of exact language in speaking and writing. From it one may derive a sense of adventure and discovery, surely an ample reward. In short, it makes a better doctor with improved technical expertise and heightened critical ability.

Criteria of a Research Problem

1. Ideally it should concern a natural phenomenon which is quantitative and preferably amenable to experimentation.

2. The subject should be capable of being stated as several alternative hypotheses. It should therefore test some proposition in which there is a real difference of opinion.

3. It may deal with some little known relationship or some neglected question. Significantly, it must arouse the curiosity and interest of the investigator.

4. The primary object is to obtain new facts in an important field, not to repeat what has been done before. We believe that the research should have some clinical application, either directly or indirectly. In the past, much purely laboratory investigation has failed for want of clinical direction and there is still much pointless research undertaken however well dressed up it appears.

5. The research project must be circumscribed, specific and quite definite in its objectives. We recommend the reading of Beveridge's (1951) 'The art of scientific investigation' and Wilson's (1952) 'An introduction to scientific research', at this stage. Claude Bernard's (1878) 'An introduction to the study of experimental medicine' is also obligatory reading.

The wise man will start a card index of possible subjects for research, and carry a small note book in his pocket in which to record ideas as they occur.

6. Finally, the research project should be adapted to the material available and be within one's capability. It is useless for anyone to plan a project which for instance, requires a great deal of histo-chemistry if he knows little of the subject and has no expert help. Learning the techniques alone may take 6–12 months, during which time the planned research has not advanced at all. Much research reviews old problems using new techniques, so that learning new techniques may be the way to open up a profitable field of discovery.

Organization

Before the research has even begun, it is vitally important to write in detail a protocol. This will in effect be a mini-paper and should set out answers to the following 8 questions:

1. What is the aim of the work?
2. How will it be achieved?
3. How will bias be eliminated?
4. What types of patients (or animals) will be studied?
5. How will the data be recorded?
6. What statistical analysis will be required?
7. Are there ethical aspects?
8. Is it likely to be worth while?

The relevant literature should be looked over fairly quickly to make sure that you do not plan to repeat what has been done success-fully before, and the protocol then discussed with an experienced colleague.

In some situations half the paper for publication has already been organized because the type of project demanded a detailed and clearly written protocol. Thus, in planning a controlled clinical trial of a new technique in management, the following questions will have had to be thought over carefully before a single patient has been treated:

1. What type of patient will be treated? What age group, and which sex?
2. How will the diagnosis of disease be made?
3. How advanced can the disease be for inclusion on the trial?
4. What is the list of exceptions or exclusions from the trial?
5. How will the controls be chosen?
6. How will the results be assessed and by whom?
7. Will it be a 'blind' or 'double blind' trial?
8. What statistical analysis will be required?

Hence, when the time comes for writing, pruning and editing is often all that is required. For advice on the conduct of clinical trials the textbook by Witts (1952) is recommended:

In other forms of research, a hypothesis may be formulated and the work then seeks new observations for its support. If it leads to a new hypothesis this in turn is tested, so that the final writing up of data may involve a series of experiments. On such occasions, the plan outlined by Trelease (1958) would seem admirable.

1. General introduction.
2. General material and methods.
3. Descriptive title of first series of experiments.
    (a) Introduction.
    (b) Materials and methods.
    (c) Experiments and results.
    (d) Discussion of results.

4. Descriptive title of second series of experiments, a, b, c, d, as before. This format can be repeated as often as necessary, finally ending with:

5. General discussion.

Two basic rules apply to writing in research:

1. Every observation and every experiment must be recorded in writing at the time they are made, preferably in a day-book so that precious data cannot be mislaid. Good note-book discipline is essential. When there is sufficient data, tables can be constructed and graphs drawn on squared paper stuck into the book. Tentative or preliminary conclusions, made perhaps after only a few experiments, should be recorded. Later, summaries of progress from a larger series of experiments will help to concentrate your thoughts and help you to be critical of your own work. If there are research-in-progress meetings at your institution, new ideas pertinent to your own projects should be written in the same book. Remember always to record the date at the top of the page whenever you write. A well documented note-book is a personal record of action, thought, and time—a precious thing. When it comes to writing the paper, direct transfer of the results from the laboratory note-book to paper without considerable editing will not produce an acceptable publication.

2. Findings should be published as soon as a significant advance in the subject has been made, and not before. To wait until all questions have been answered and all possible hypotheses explored may take a life-time. To man no end is discoverable. Everything is relative; nothing is certain. The technique of writing for publication differs little from that outlined in Chapters 1 and 2, but we would point out that much research is written up too quickly. It is stupid to believe that research which has taken two years to complete can be written satisfactorily in two weeks (Fig. 8).

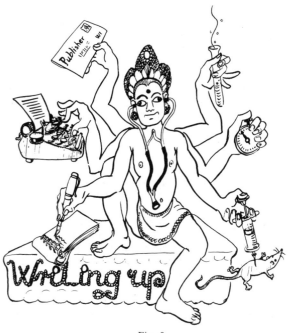

Fig. 8.

6. Synopsis for a Learned Society

Some day you may wish to present a paper to a scientific society of your choice. Such meetings may be popular and the programme over-subscribed. To overcome the difficulties in the selection of papers offered, several societies now demand a synopsis beforehand; these are then judged by a panel of experts and the final selection made. All this means that however good a speaker you may be and however brilliant your work, in the beginning you are only a paper candidate. If you cannot set out well a synopsis of what you wish to present, you may never have the opportunity to speak.

How then can one overcome the first hurdle and have the work approved? There are 7 stages in its production:

1. The first thing to do is to read carefully the regulations most societies provide for applicants. If the abstract is limited to 200 words it is foolish to exceed the total; it is also unwise to condense it to less than half the allowed volume in case the assessor should think that you have really very little to say. If the regulations specify no more than two references, it is ridiculous to give half-a-dozen; they do not impress anyone.

2. To succeed, the writer must know his purpose. This should be evident from the title, but if it is not then it must be quite clear from the script.

3. To succeed, the writer must write for someone, for a specific audience who will understand his subject anyway. At this stage he has to please the expert; to interest is to inform. One detail is worth a thousand generalizations, and such phrases as 'a series of patients was examined', and 'future management will be discussed' are valueless.

4. The synopsis requires a structure. The introduction need only be one sentence but the main message must contain the factual and significant results of the work. The conclusions can be written in one sentence or one paragraph but their validity should appear reasonable from the data presented. Since tables are usually not accepted, condensation is always required.

5. Make every word count so that you are economical of words yet the information given is quite specific. Hence revision of the script is always necessary. Give the references some impact too by recording the most important and by omitting those which show clearly that you have little new to contribute because it has all been published before.

6. If the spoken contribution is to be limited to 10 minutes,

writing on a subject which will clearly take much longer to put over is foolish. It may be better to deal with diagnosis or treatment and not to attempt to squeeze in both.

7. The synopsis should always be typed in double spacing, the format required by the society accepted, and the correct number of copies dispatched. Rejection carries no stigma. If you think that your subject is important and the synopsis informative, it should be submitted for the following meeting. After all, there is only limited time available at every meeting to hear a dissertation on one of the many advances that are occurring in medicine.

7. Speaking after the Publication

Having written a paper and had it published you may then be invited to give a lecture on the subject. The paper written for publication is a poor basis for the proposed lecture; hasty editing and slides from the illustrations, appears to be all that is required. This is not so. A lecture requires:

1. A new script, not the paper abbreviated.
2. New illustrations, not from the published paper.

Both the script and the illustrations must be tailored to the occasion and to the audience. Adequate time will have to be allowed for preparation and practice, and we have discussed this at length elsewhere (Calnan and Barabas, 1972). If you wish to write well then develop a love for literature, and read it. If you wish to speak well, listen to good speakers on the radio or at public lectures. Learning to speak well is a life-long process; it can be pleasurable and brings its own reward of a job well done. Standards formed only from the second rate will be second rate, so watch the art. The author who embarks on a lecture unthinkingly may destroy the reputation he has gained by writing. In speaking you will have to:

1. capture the attention of your audience from the beginning;
2. state your objectives clearly;

3. eliminate details which may confuse, and concentrate only on new concepts;

4. discuss the purpose of the work and the conclusions drawn from it;

5. use slides of less complexity than the illustrations from the published paper.

But this subject is large and we advise you to consult, 'Speaking at Medical Meetings' (1972).

8. Publishing after the Lecture

If an editor asks to publish a successful lecture you may have given, some alteration will be necessary to tidy up the script, and make the work valuable to a larger and unknown reading public. If you wish to publish results of some new scientific work, having already spoken about it, then we advise a completely new script.

Modifications of the original lecture rarely appear well in print; that humorous and brilliant introduction for the lecture becomes trite in the publication. There will be need to give details of the methods used, and more explicit tables of the results, with the relevant statistics. You may beguile your listeners with fine words and poor facts in a lecture, but not in the written account where the reader can go over the words again and check what you have stated. Facts speak for themselves and without them scientific writing is nothing.

9. Consulting the Library

If there is a medical library in your institution or nearby and you do not know it well, take time to browse around (Fig. 9). Find out how books and periodicals are arranged and try to evaluate the library's merits and deficits; there will be both. Consult the expert, the librarian, by stating what you want to do and allow some of your enthusiasm for the subject to brush off on to her. If she has been helpful in finding references you can say 'thank-you' very simply by acknowledging this aid at the end of your paper; send her two reprints when it is published, one for herself and the other for submission with any future application for promotion. This is no more than good manners and is generally appreciated.

One should talk to colleagues working in the same field for help in finding a lead into the relevant literature. If a drug is involved,

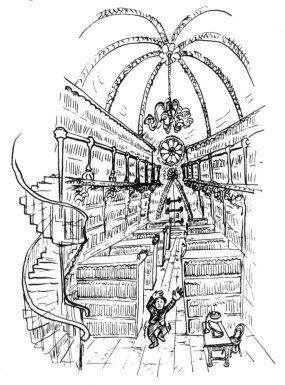

Fig. 9.

43

pharmaceutical companies will usually provide references and re-prints. It is also necessary to be familiar with essential sources of information:

Text books, Encyclopaedias, Dictionaries.
Review journals, monographs.
Index medicus.
Year books and the Medical Annual.

We recommend that any author who is interested in making the most use of his library should read and digest 'How to use a library' by L. T. Morton (1968). When asking the librarian's help remember to:

1. Allow enough time for her to obtain the text you want, if it has to be obtained on inter-library loan.

2. Verify everything. Don't accept a reference from a text book as accurate; there is more than a 10% chance that it will be wrong.

3. When looking for references, sharpen the question you ask by deciding on the years of publication and in what language you wish to search.

4. Discriminate in what you read. There is no need to read every article on the subject; it is equally important to know when to stop. Reading does not make a man wise; it only makes him learned.

Recording References

Medical writing is a multidisciplined and sophisticated act if you wish to do it well. You should therefore cultivate the habit of reading journals regularly and recording immediately the essential findings on cards.

1. The method by which this is done is not explicit, but we recom-mend that 20 × 13 cm cards be carried at all times. These should be ruled on one side only, for the essential reference and plain at the back for notes of detail. diagrams, and tables.

2. The lay-out should always be the same and in general we advise the Harvard system. Leave the top line of the cards blank for key-words to be inserted later, depending on how you wish to file them.

The author's names and initials should be written on the second line on the left side, and on the right the year of publication. On the third line in the middle of the card, record the journal, volume number, with first and last pages. Add the month of issue for easy referral later. Beneath this write correctly the exact title.

At the bottom left make your own assessment of the value of the paper as 'good, bad, or non-informative' and a note on the type of illustrations and any list of references given.

3. Each card may now be filed in a box and arranged in alphabetical order. On the lid of the box one can record the title of the subject, such as, 'Venous thrombosis'. The dividing cards can be labelled sequentially as, (a) 'Venous thrombosis—causes', (b) 'Treatment', (c) 'Prevention', and so on. Many of the reference cards will cover more than one aspect of your personal subdivisions and will have to be filed in the most appropriate section. However, since all cards are filed in one box it is probably less labour to look through other sections than to make out cross-index cards.

4. When your paper has been written, the list of references will be easy to compose. Just pull out each card as required, arrange them in alphabetical order and write one new card only as an example to the typist of the style in which the journal prefers to list them. There is still no uniformity in journals and until there is, we believe that the Harvard system is the simplest for personal note taking.

5. Cards should also be made out for your own papers as they are published. If they are filed in a separate section, you now have a basis for drawing up the annual report of your unit, with little effort.

6. If you always carry a dozen cards in your jacket pocket, you are constantly equipped to record information from reading, as well as noting the names of interesting patients. The cards should also record reprints, photocopies and articles torn out of journals, with a note of where these can be found in your office. If you have a box-file marked 'Administration' a paper on surgical technique might be usefully filed there because it also dealt with the organization in the operating theatre, a subject with which you are concerned.

7. One evening once a month looking through your cards is time

well spent, for thinking out new ideas and for rearrangement of your collection. You may decide that you have to cover the literature more widely and the only way to do this is by consulting a central agency, such as the Medlars Service.

A Computer Search

This is commonly called a Medlars Search (Medical literature analysis and retrieval system) and details can be obtained from 'The U.K. Medlars Service, National Lending Library, Boston Spa, Yorkshire, LS23 7BQ'. A handbook for users is also available. The titles of about 2800 journals (or 165 000 articles per year) are held on tape and the computer will select and print out those you require. However there are snags, and it is too easy to be burdened with many hundreds of titles for which you have no use.

1. The decision to use Medlars must be made after examining all journals available, and after consulting the librarian.
2. The search must be strictly confined—by years of publication, language and the correct keyword (see Medical Subjects index, Me SH). If you wish to consult papers on wound healing (an enormous subject in itself) you will probably not benefit from a paper on wounds, written entirely in Japanese. Key-words can often be located by noting the headings and subheadings used in the Index Medicus. Recent papers by Thornton (1971) and Barber, Barraclough, and Gray (1972), should also be consulted.

10. Co-authors

A time will come when the publication reports the work of a team. Who should be an author? This is a more difficult question to answer than at first appears. If it is customary for the name of the senior man to appear on all publications from the department then he must read all, correct and comment; but on the whole this is little short of piracy.

Alexander (1953) believed that the essential requisite for author-ship of a scientific paper was the contribution of creative thinking, and asked, 'How often is it the product of 6–8 individuals thinking in unison?' The current practice of multiple authorship undoubtedly stems from the growth of research teams. When there are multiple authors, one man only must write the paper. Multiple writers produce a patchwork of different styles. To allow each to write a section is ridiculous!

Creative thinking should not be confused with expert consultation. Our own rule is that an author must have contributed something worth while. If he has only corrected the typescript or given advice this can be acknowledged at the end of the paper.

1. Authors arranged in alphabetical order, should all have contributed equally to the work.

2. The first name on the list implies that he has done the greatest amount of work and other names are arranged then in proportion.

3. If there are only two names, the first has probably done the work and the other has written it.

4. If there are only two authors, the senior may elect to go second even though there has been equal contribution, because the advantage may be greater for the junior. In the next paper, in a continuing study, the senior man can be the first author to redress the balance.

5. Commonly the senior's name comes last, by convention, where contributors are equal and multiple.

6. If the contribution is likely to be part of a thesis for one of the authors, then his name should be the first whenever possible; he will probably have done most of the work anyway. If this order is not observed it may jeopardize the validity of the thesis as being essentially a personal project.

3

THE CONSULTANT

'People ask you for criticism, but they only want praise'
Somerset Maugham

Essential writing for a consultant usually means all those jobs which cannot be delegated successfully to others, yet includes such papers on his own work which he particularly wishes to write.

The consultant's motives for writing may have changed from those he had as a junior. Success is still just as necessary, but the driving force, the desire for publication in a learned journal is not enough. He may wish for payment, not only as a reward for labour but because payment provides a basis of comparison and shows that his work has value in a competitive market. Prestige, too, and writing for response (though he will have done that for research funds) are other motives. Finally, there is writing for pleasure—the sheer joy of composing a neat piece, of formulating abstract ideas, of converting the complex into intelligible prose, of wrestling with words to construct a harmony of sense and sound. The change in outlook towards writing may have been imperceptible or deliberate, but change there is.

For vivid wr'ting an educated man probably needs 30 000 words at his command, including all those specialized medical terms learned during training. But your readers may know only 3000 so what can you do? If you wish to keep your writing trim and attractive, simple terms, simple constructions, and only a small mixture of polysyllables are essential ingredients. Each word in a sentence must carry its weight and all those which don't say anything must be erased. Unfortunately, with seniority in position and years, the lure of the magic of words and the desire to use the more showy qualities of the language, increases. The temptation should be resisted, otherwise later re-reading of your own prose will be nothing to be proud of.

1. Coaching

If he is fortunate enough still to be in a position to make original observations, to carry through a piece of laboratory research, to devise a new procedure, or to be recognized as a pioneer with grey hair, the consultant will have picked up an accomplice on the way. When it comes to reporting, who should write the paper? The obvious choice is the consultant who may have published many papers already. But this is wrong. The consultant has a duty to his co-author, to teach him the craft of writing.

The act of writing, like surgical technique, has to be learned the hard way—by practice. As a co-author the junior should be required to write the paper. The consultant's job in this, as in many other instances when he is asked to vet a paper for publication by any other junior doctor, is to lead the writer towards good prose and accurate, factual reporting.

If your assistant has written a script, then 80% of the work has been done. The fact that the remaining 20% seems hard labour is unimportant. Correct the carbon copy and ask him to retain the top copy for future reference: it will serve as a humble reminder in years to come when he has become a polished author in his own right, of how bad his writing was at that time. But corrections are not easy. You have to know (and you should know by then) the temperament of your co-author, and how far you can go without pushing him to despair. Gentleness and firmness are essential qualities. If the English is a bit rough, try not to be too finicky and pedantic in your corrections. He is developing a style which, in a new age, may have more appeal than yours. The important thing is to make it appear a joint effort, which requires tact and a great deal of patience.

The other individual to watch is the man who has made original discoveries which should be recorded, but who has no desire to put pen to paper. It is the duty of a consultant to advise and encourage him otherwise. This may not be easy, but then many things in life are thus. A tentative outline of the script, many conversations, and even a glass of sherry at the appropriate time help to change a negative attitude. To fire enthusiasm is always possible and the reward is often memorable. Our own view is that authorship, like so many acquired skills, must start early in life. The consultant who encourages his junior to report an interesting or unusual patient, by helping with the references, picking out the best photographs, finding the most suitable journal, and declining recognition in the final article, has done a creditable job.

2. Reporting a Conference

Medical writing for money usually means a chapter in a book, or a review article for the lay press. These works are commissioned by the editor, who may alter what you have written. Another source of useful finance comes when you are to attend an important meeting in some distant part of the world, for journals are prepared to pay for a report on the proceedings. To be successful some of the methods of newspaper reporters have to be adopted.

1. Since you will have the detailed programme in advance of the meeting, it is worth trying to pick out the news items. You should not attempt to report on everything because the publication which follows most international meetings will do that. The object is to select what is new or controversial and concentrate on providing a clear, detailed summary. It is wise to look up the speakers in a medical directory before you go and hence know something of their positions and interests. Big names on the programme may attract participants but their owners may often have little new to contribute.

2. Speed is essential, so if you intend to have a beach holiday afterwards, the copy has to be run off first. It will need to be typed and mailed to the editor quickly, for few subjects in medicine are new and topical for long. The length of the report should have been agreed beforehand, and it is important to keep within this limit. If the editor has predicted a date for publication you may have to arrange an address to which the proofs can be sent.

Having written papers for status and personal advancement for a number of years, it is nice to find people are prepared to pay for your literary efforts. But you must do it well.

3. An Editorial

Some people can write good editorials, others never learn the art. An editorial is rather like an aerial view of a landscape (Fig. 10). The essential features are picked out, put into correct perspective and the writer's personal vantage point is subdued. To compose a good editorial requires more than good literary style and practice in writing short essays. Expert knowledge, a sense of history and complete impartiality are essential. An ability to look into the future is an

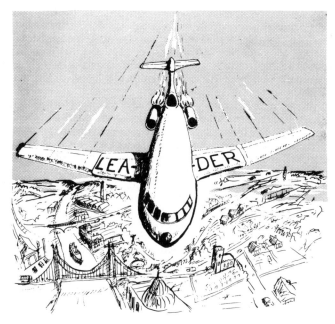

Fig. 10.

advantage, for what you write may stimulate others to future research—speculation has a very special place. An editorial should:

1. be factual and informative;
2. state a problem as an hypothesis;
3. collect all recent and relevant data about it;
4. weigh the data to determine its value and application to the problem;
5. frame alternative hypotheses;
6. select the solution which appears the best and most logical;
7. exhort the reader to act.

An editorial is a piece of professional writing. The best will be clear and readable, argumentative, imperative, abrasive, and conciliatory, all within 200–400 words. The good editorial raises controversy among its readers and may provoke spontaneous and often emotional reaction in the correspondence columns of the same journal.

In medicine a single disease or a method of treatment for a group of diseases may form the subject of an editorial written by an expert in the field. The title or heading is usually dispensed by the chief editor and sometimes appears unrelated to the text; eye-catching phrases are more important than exactitudes. Such editorials can provide a survey of contemporary thought and practice, for generalizations have to be stated; there is no place for tables and graphs. They also provide material for historical reviews, so that if you wish to know what people thought about, say, cancer of the colon, 20 years ago, an editorial written then will tell you a great deal, including references to the important literature.

If you are asked to write an editorial you will have to discuss with the editor:

1. the total number of words;
2. the exact subject—diagnosis or treatment. You must be quite clear what you want to achieve;
3. the period to be surveyed;

4. the language of the literature to be scanned;

5. the date by which your copy must be in his hands;

6. the examination of papers submitted recently, and which are intended to be included in the same issue of the journal.

4. Reviewing a Book

A reviewer's lot is not a happy one. He must have knowledge of the subject, yet will find difficulty in hiding his own contrary views without appearing conceited. The job cannot be delegated to a junior for it requires the highest levels of accomplishment and interpretive skills, so it has to be fitted into a busy practice. The demands of scholarship are high and the time expended large (Roland, 1971).

There are literary rewards, however, because the opportunity to review a book offers a chance to write well, to be creative and to develop a personal style; it is not the opportunity for cleverness but for good powerful writing and a nice turn of phrase. By way of preparation, we recommend the reading of professional reviews of the theatre, music and literature which are published in the major daily newspapers. From these may be learnt the art of vivid reporting in few words. The Lancet and the British Medical Journal carry book reviews each week, of different style and calibre; usually 200–500 words are ample for the purpose.

There are certain rules to be observed by the medical reviewer.

1. Read the whole work with perception.

2. Be sympathetic towards the author, who may have taken a great deal of trouble for more than a year, to set down on paper a difficult subject.

3. Listing the contents is not the job of the reviewer unless in themselves they are unusual or unexpected from the title. The price is commonly included in the title of the review: if you consider the book to be value for money, say so.

4. Note the syntax, punctuation and style of the book, and try to answer 8 questions:

Does it cover what the author intended?
Whom was it written for?
Is it easily readable and is it factual?
Is it informative?
Is the main message clear?
Are the illustrations good?
Is the binding attractive?
Is it worth the price?

On the answers to these the reviewer can base his recommendation to others to purchase the book.

5. The review should synthesize and analyse the work of the author in a neat summary. Such appraisal is the essence of competent reviewing. It is not easy. Criticism can of course be explicit or implicit, and a few well chosen phrases can lift or damn a piece of work. The style can be personal or impersonal, but it must be authoritative; the wide knowledge of the reviewer can with advantage come through.

5. A Thesis

Writing a thesis is a major undertaking. To be accepted it must report new work and comply with the University regulations. The first thing to do therefore is to request the necessary regulations, to read them carefully, and, if in any doubt about their interpretation, to consult an official for clarification. Many universities insist on the candidates having a supervisor; he should be chosen with care so that he knows your subject sufficiently to give good advice and has time enough to devote his whole attention to regular consultations.

To be successful is a different matter. Without self-discipline and hard thinking it cannot be done! Without enthusiasm it becomes a dull chore, which shows in the writing. There must be sufficient time to carry the project through, perhaps three years of part-time effort or one year of full-time work depending on the degree. Some take longer, but if after five years the thesis has not been completed it should probably be abandoned. The thesis is an educational tool. It is the result of one individual's work and should present a formal statement as an hypothesis, preferably with more than one approach to the topic. It should present all the data obtained in the study; it also offers the opportunity for an extended and argumentative discussion. It is meant to be a scholarly dissertation. A thesis, however, does not have to be lengthy to be erudite, and in our view, most are too long and make tedious reading; size and quality do not go hand in hand (Fig. 11).

We presume that preliminary explorative work has already been done on the proposed subject, and that a protocol of the definitive project has been written. The candidate should choose his own subject. It should be one in which he is already interested, and better still, one for which he has already carried out a great deal of work. He should have had some experience of writing and of the principles of research. In choosing a subject one has to be especially wary of the ideas which seem the most self-evident and the most obvious; they are current and we have heard them accepted as truisms from early days. Yet it is exactly these ideas which should be examined more closely as the basis for an exciting thesis.

It helps to remember that there are 6 stages in the preparation of a thesis.

1. Early Planning

Right at the beginning, a précis of the work should be written on two sheets of paper. This brief outline may be submitted with the application to the university for approval to proceed. Because the thesis will be a study in depth, the title demands particular attention; it should be well defined and well confined. You must be clear about the problem under discussion and why you selected this one for study.

A great deal of reading will have to be done, and relevant findings should be made on 15 × 10 cm record cards, together with the exact reference. Reading should be selective and perceptive. It is a truism that good writing follows good reading and the wider the

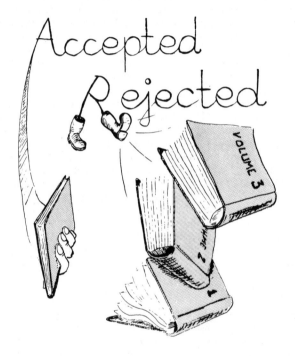

Fig. 11.

variety, the wider the general approach to the subject. The candidate is expected to know all the resources of a library and the best guide is to enlist the help of the medical librarian. It is usually impossible to review all the literature, so you have to use judgement. In the same way, if statistics will feature in the finished work, the advice of the statistician must be sought at an early stage.

Finally, ideas should be recorded on paper within the recognised structure for the finished work. Some universities lay down precise details for the lay out, binding and the general format. To some extent the structure depends on the work reported and it is advisable to look over successful theses of similar nature. In any case, many subheadings will be needed to make it readable. Few theses flow like a well written novel.

A possible analytical outline might be:

1. Title page, with name, degrees and date of submission.
2. The curriculum vitae of the candidate.
3. Abstract of the work, of about 50 words or so.
4. Summary of the main findings, perhaps 400–600 words.
5. Survey of the relevant published work, described in depth. This should not be a chronological list from earliest times, but a well-considered account strictly limited by the title. This introduction should be no more than one quarter of the whole thesis.
6. Materials and methods.
7. Patients studied.
8. Results, in chronological order and in order of complexity. Tables, graphs, diagrams, will all be included in this section which should form the major portion of the script.
9. Discussion, that is what you set out to do and what was found. Sub-headings will be essential when changing from one topic to the next. If you mix your own data with other published work, utter confusion will follow.
10. Conclusion.
11. References.
12. Acknowledgements.
13. Appendices for detailed data which if retained within the text would impede the flow and rhythm of the script. These may be tables, case reports, or special analytical techniques.

An alternative structure more suited to work which has included several experiments of a different nature would be:

1–4. As before.
5. General introduction.
6. Experiment I (a) Materials and methods.
           (b) Results.
           (c) Discussion and Conclusions.
7. Experiment II (a) Material and methods.
           (b) Results.
           (c) Discussion and conclusions.
   This sub-structure can be repeated as often as required.
8. General discussion of results.
10–12. As before.

Each section heading should be written on a separate sheet of paper, to receive notes of data and ideas. During this period of assimilation it is advisable to purchase a box file 27 × 36 × 8 cm into which are placed all scraps of paper with bright ideas, library reference cards, cuttings from journals, reprints, preliminary data, and notes recording conversations with colleagues.

2. Definitive Planning

One day when you have a couple of hours of quiet, empty all the contents of the box file on to a large table. Now is the time to sort over what you have acquired and to decide whether the thesis is possible, or even likely within the time available.

The definitive research may have only just begun. Even so it should become clear by now what aspects of the subject will be the most demanding in time and effort.

3. Preliminary Writing

At this stage the project should be going well. Now is the time to start getting fit to write well. Start writing the introduction, material and methods, some results and part of the discussion. There will be gaps of course for not all the data will yet be available. During this time, leisure hours should be spent in reading good English, the influence of which will be noted in better writing later. Good reading is intellectual nourishment, as important to the candidate in producing a scholarly work as the data on which the thesis is based. Everyone writing a thesis must cultivate some literary values, an important part of the exercise. The manuscript should not be typed at this stage but written in long-hand leaving plenty of space for corrections.

4. Handling the Data

As each set of experiments is completed, tables should be constructed. Examination of the results in this form should indicate to the candidate what new work may have to be done to support the original hypothesis or to substantiate the likely conclusions. A thesis which proves everything and explains nothing is hardly meritorious; critical analysis in interpretation is mandatory.

5. Writing

As soon as the work has been completed, it is wise to take one or two weeks leave to write and assemble the whole thesis in one session. By doing so, continuity of thought, unity of composition, flow and readability, are likely to be assured. This stage is undoubtedly hard work and the most difficult physical act to undertake. But it has to be done. The thesis has now been written, an ample reward for the effort.

6. Revision, Rewriting, Binding, Submission

After the torrid atmosphere of the previous stage, revision is almost an anticlimax. The wise man will wait at least a month before revising his script, so that it can be examined as though it were a new work. Revision and rewriting can be taken at a gentle pace. Most theses can be improved by skilful editing: many are rejected because they are badly written. They do not do justice to the facts they contain.

The work should be read to answer three questions:

(a) Is the logic correct?
(b) If the logic is sound, are the basic assumptions at fault?
(c) Are the conclusions justified from the evidence presented?

If the answers are 'yes', apply the rules of good English, examining each paragraph at first and then sentence by sentence. Prune relentlessly (Fig. 12) until the manuscript is to your entire satisfaction.

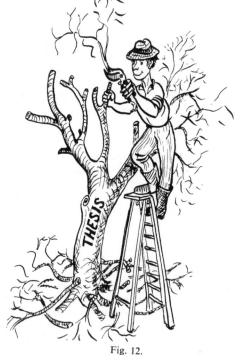

Fig. 12.

Finally, have it typed and read this version for errors. The value of the thesis lies not so much in the quality of the work done but rather in the personal discipline which has been acquired.

In all instances, three persons should be allowed to read the final script:

1. The Head of your Department, who may be one of the university's assessors. It is embarrassing for both of you if he has had no prior knowledge of the work.

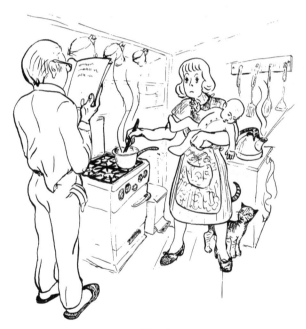

Fig. 13.

2. Your supervisor, who may not have had the opportunity to see the completed work in final form.

3. A friend, or colleague, or if possible your wife (Fig. 13), to assess the literary quality and clarity of the writing. Even if their opinions may lead to further revisions and corrections, the gain is usually rewarding.

A good rule is not to publish any detail from the thesis before it is submitted to the university. Once the degree has been awarded, parts of the work can be submitted to the journal of choice but will require rewriting. If the work is so important that some aspect should be published early, to establish the claim of priority, then it is essential that the candidate's name be first when there are multiple authors.

6. A Monograph

The technique for writing a monograph for publication is much the same as for a thesis—but with one big difference: the end product must be a commercial proposition. You therefore have to ask such searching questions as, 'Who am I writing for?' 'Who will buy the book?'. Most theses are not saleable however good-looking the cover.

The lay-out of a monograph will be quite different and much of the scientific data compressed and simplified. Editing a thesis usually will not do. The whole has to be rewritten with quite a different slant.

B. THE CRAFT

4

PREPARING TO WRITE

'I have collected a mass of facts, ideas, experience, but I cannot yet arrange them into any system or order them into a definite pattern'—
Somerset Maugham

1. The Ground Plan, Flow Chart, and Title

In order to write a paper for publication you must have something worthwhile to report. The significant paper requires a great deal of preparation, knowledge of the mechanics of writing, and a basic structure or form.

A paper on a scientific subject has a beginning, a middle and an end. The basic structure is commonly as follows, and although many consider it unduly restrictive, no better method has been evolved for routine use. In planning and organization we are concerned here with principles rather than detail.

A. The Conventional Structure

I.	Introduction	Holds the reader's attention—the how, why, what when, where and who?
		States the problem and reasons for the investigation in simple terms.
II.	Material	Who, what, why?
III.	Methods	Experimental technique.
		Experimental design.
		Methods of assay. Protocol of assessment.
IV.	Results	Separates fact from opinion. As Marcus Aurelius wrote: 'Treat with respect the power you have to form an opinion'—and don't muddle it up with fact.
V.	Discussion	1. Of the work presented: introduces no new facts.

2. Of the work related to that of others.

3. Of its relation to other concepts.

VI. Conclusion 1. It confirms what everyone knows.

2. It confirms what people have suspected.

3. It's new and has never been thought of before.

VII. Summary This is what will be read first and abstracted so it should be factual and informative.

VIII. Illustrations, tables, and legends.

IX. References to the literature cited.

Use the format proscribed by the journal, but personally we prefer the Harvard system—name, initials, year of publication, journal, volume, page. Add the exact wording of the title if the journal specifies this requirement (and in the language of origin).

X. Acknowledgements for diagrams, photography, technical help.

B. The Short Structure (for a minor presentation)

I. Introduction.

II. Methods of study.

III. Results.

IV. Discussion and conclusions.

V. References.

Structure is the bare skeleton on which to hang, by creative writing, ideas, data, inferences and conclusions. If the work is presented in this way it now has form, is interesting and may become not just good reading but an important reference for the future.

It is an advantage to write the general theme on a single piece of paper so that it can be viewed as a whole. If a coherent story can be written in say 200 words then there will be little difficulty later.

For the conventional structure obtain 7 sheets of paper each with its own title at the top, such as 'Introduction', 'Material', as from the master plan. Even at this stage two additional sheets will be required for 'references' and 'acknowledgements' even though there may be little to write on them.

On each sheet write brief indications of experiments, facts, thoughts, and observations which are considered appropriate to the heading. Then examine the sheets and ask yourself three questions:

1. Is the item necessary?
2. Is it in the correct section?
3. Are all necessary items included?

At this stage the concept of a paper has taken some shape, but there has been no attempt to write it. It should become clear to you at this stage whether the paper is worth writing at all. If there is doubt, the question can be asked again at the next stage of preparation after tables and figures have been constructed.

We can now construct a flow chart of the events which must follow.

The Ground Plan or Flow Chart

Collect the data.
↓
Write the title, authors, and look at the proposed journal.
↓
Outline the theme on one sheet of paper.
↓
Transfer to 9 separate sheets.
↓
Consult library references.
↓
Make out tables. Collect graphs, charts and other illustrations.
↓
Rearrange notes.
↓

67

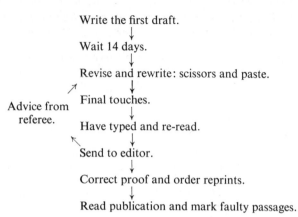

Write the first draft.

↓

Wait 14 days.

↓

Revise and rewrite: scissors and paste.

↓

Final touches.

↓

Advice from referee.

Have typed and re-read.

↓

Send to editor.

↓

Correct proof and order reprints.

↓

Read publication and mark faulty passages.

It looks a lot but really there are no short cuts; an author is assessed by the quality of the paper turned out, not by the amount of work that went into it. The next step is to specify the title of the proposed paper.

The Title

The exact title of the proposed paper should be written out on a separate sheet of paper. By so doing at this early stage it will define and limit the field in which you are going to write. The title should be chosen with care; it will be indexed by agencies (such as Index Medicus, Current Contents) and libraries all over the world, and influences others with similar interests to read your paper.

1. The title should be as informative as possible and should state exactly what you mean.

2. It should be as short as possible. If there are too many 'key-words' in the title, the paper may be indexed under several headings in different abstracting journals: there may thus be excessive demands for reprints by persons hoping to read something of particular interest to them. However, the essential key-word must be in the title.

68

3. The title should be specific and accurate. It should have punch, that is it should convey the maximum information with the minimum of words. Asher (1972) entitled one essay 'Myxoedematous madness' —this is far better than 'Certain psychotic features observed in patients with low protein-bound iodine'.

4. The title should be reconsidered again when the paper is finished. The contest for the best title is between man (the author) and machine (the indexing agency). If you wish to know how ambiguous and funny some titles can be, consult any issue of the 'Journal of irreproducible results'.

2. Assembly

If structure is strategy then here we deal with tactics, the art of disposition. The first thing is to prepare illustrations before any writing is done at all. This phase of organization is important and will further clarify how the paper will be written (Fig. 14).

There are 5 important steps in treating the data from an investigation.

1. Make out tables and check all calculations.

2. Draw graphs to show relationships. Plot them even if they will not be published.

3. Examine written notes for sufficient detail and make out headings and sub-headings as initial guides. If the paper is long they can be retained to help the reader.

4. State the conclusions. Do they explain the facts? It may be necessary to verify some by more tests. Look for all the possible conclusions and do not emphasize only one.

5. Look for exceptions. Record and check their value and ask why the expected result was not obtained.

In writing, order is everything. One has to marshal the facts in their correct sequence, to discriminate between what is of primary and what is of secondary importance, and to develop an analytical mind. According to MacPhail (1911) there are three kinds of writers: those who never think at all, those who think only as they write, and

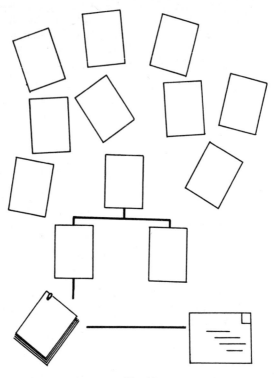

Fig. 14.

those who have thought before taking a pen in the hand. We have
time only for the last for there is a two-way relationship between
writing and thinking. Good writing is impossible without clear
thinking; careful writing assists logical thought because it clarifies,
sharpens and demarcates thought.

3. Illustrations

The term illustration has a wide embracing meaning. The results and conclusions are also illustrations but in abstract form, but here we will limit the term to material which is not text—tables, graphs, diagrams, drawings, and photographs.

Illustrations are international in character for they are not modified by language or custom. Combined with mathematics, graphs, diagrams, and charts can convey information readily (Fig. 15).

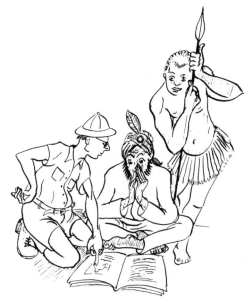

Fig. 15.

Illustrations also break up the text into smaller portions which may thus be digested more easily. If well done, they are invaluable but their main purpose is to throw light on obscure or difficult material and not to beautify a text.

There are 10 important rules for the inclusion of illustrations in any publication:

1. The illustration must convey information. There is an old proverb which states that 'one picture is worth 1000 words'; We have seen illustrations which require nearly that number of words by way of explanation.

2. It should attract the reader and enable him to grasp the message of the paper more easily. It may thus clarify those parts of the text which might be misconstrued otherwise.

3. All illustrations must be an integral part of the treatise, and entirely relevant. They either augment the treatise or convey extra information with little or no text; hence, some mathematical and chemical formulae are best presented as illustrations.

4. The good illustration does not repeat information adequately presented in the text. If it does, it is superfluous and should be omitted.

5. Tables and graphs should neither duplicate nor contradict each other.

6. An illustration should have impact—to introduce, to explain, or to summarize the data.

7. A well-designed illustration is often recollected and may remind the reader of the vital message when the text has long been forgotten.

8. Illustrations must contain all the information the reader can be expected to require, and not more than can be assimilated within the time at his disposal. It must be appropriate for the expected audience. A complicated electrical diagram suitable for an engineering journal is out of place in a general medical or surgical publication.

9. If more than one illustration is being used, retain the same format, lettering, and general appearance in each.

10. In all art work, simplicity is the keynote. Secondary detail should be omitted from tables, graphs and diagrams. Finally, remember that readers often photocopy a paper for their files instead of asking the author for a reprint. But photographs and half-tone

illustrations do not copy well, whereas line drawings reproduce faithfully.

A. Tables

Tables should be completely intelligible to others and have three objectives:

1. To allow the reader to glean the content of the work from them, without even reading the text. One should avoid undue complexity in tables and illustrations for the object is to reveal their purpose and results at a glance (Fig. 16). If there is a choice of tables or graph then

Table

Experimental Lymphoedema

Common iliac vein blood flow in ml/min/Kg. body weight

Means and Standard Deviations in 9 Dogs

Time	Normal leg	Swollen leg	Significance t test
1 month	9·0 (1·03)	24·8 (2·61)	$P < 0·01$
3 months	10·9 (0·87)	16·5 (2·31)	$P < 0·05$
Significance t test	Nil	$P < 0·01$	

Fig. 16.

ask yourself if trends are more important to the reader than exact values. Rarely both are equally essential.

2. To provide an extended synopsis of the proposed text.

3. To allow the matching of data in tables with the items in each

73

section to show if the conclusions are justified. They therefore permit one to decide at an early stage whether the script outline should be modified, abandoned, or some further work done. Hence time will not be wasted in writing a paper which will never see daylight. At this stage tables are of two kinds:

(i) private, to help the author to write clearly and convincingly;
(ii) public, for inclusion in the final paper.

Tables often constitute the entire evidence put forward to support the conclusions, and therefore require careful planning. They should later be examined for inconsistencies and redundancies.

Rules for Tables

1. Each table should be a single unit of communication, completely informative in itself. The completeness of a table depends on common sense.

2. A table must supply the maximum of information so that the text can be shorter and more precise. It must be referred to in the text, but should be typed on a separate sheet.

3. It can show the results of experiments, but the simple transfer of recordings directly from the laboratory notebook is not good enough; they have to be pruned and arranged in the correct order.

4. A table should present numbers which can be compared with work already published. The units of measurement must be clearly stated.

5. Each table requires at the top a well thought out title which announces its purpose. Column headings should be independent of the text, and items must be grouped logically so that normal and control values are close together. Each table should be set out so that it makes only one point and leads to only one conclusion.

6. The shape of the table depends on the lay-out of the journal chosen for publication. It can be long or broad depending on a one or two column format in the journal. We advise that all tables be rotated through 90° to see if they present the data better that way.

7. Tables are expensive to print, and if large, may be difficult to

understand. Condensation can be achieved by dropping unimportant values and by eliminating unnecessary words.

B. Diagrams

The preliminary examination of most data is facilitated by the use of diagrams. Diagrams prove nothing but do bring outstanding features readily to the eye. They need not be elegant. They are valuable in suggesting critical tests to be applied to the collected data, and perhaps in explaining the conclusions founded on them; they have, therefore, an important place in the formation of a worthwhile publication (Fig. 17).

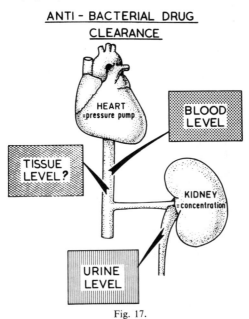

Fig. 17.

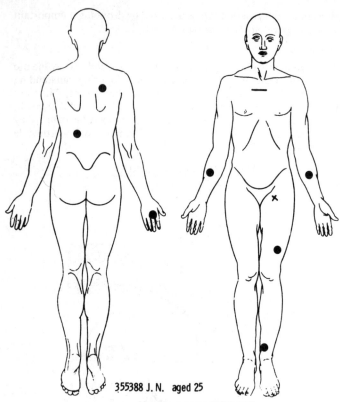

355388 J. N.   aged 25

24 moles removed 1969-1971
7 malignant melanoma
9 junctional naevi

Fig. 18.

76

In addition, rough sketches will relieve some of the physical effort in composing the prose. They act as a personal aid, as a visual stimulus, to clear writing. If they are found to be important then the rough diagram can be handed to the professional artist after the completion of the first draft. In some instances a printed body outline will convey information quickly, whereas the more elaborate artist's sketch may not (Fig. 18).

The value of diagrams lies in the capacity to:

1. aid intelligibility of the paper; they are particularly useful for illustrating apparatus and directions of flow in fluid systems;
2. provide an economy of words in the script (Fig. 19);

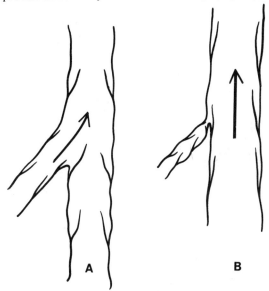

A   B

Fig. 19.

3. present definitive ideas in an artistic medium;

4. influence the script so that they can be modified or omitted as writing proceeds;

5. allow the substitution of a photograph or table, whichever is the more appropriate in the final version. It is important to note that diagrams and script are often mutually exclusive. Choose one or the other, not both.

6. crystallize one concept even though the textual description may be adequate (Fig. 20).

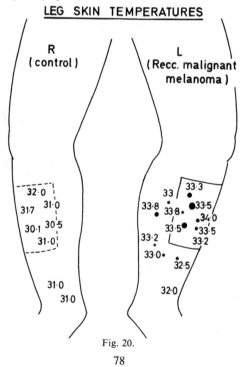

Fig. 20.

78

The author who is also an amateur artist may wish to sketch his own diagrams. If well done they add a certain charm to the text. They should be drawn in pencil and completed in waterproof black India ink. We suggest that they are then photocopied, which helps to show up any faults in technique, and used during the writing of the paper. Half-plate glossy prints are submitted to the editor, not the originals.

An engineering drawing that is orthographic or isometric should be drawn specially to include the information needed and nothing more. Exploded diagrams are useful tools but should be examined critically before inclusion with the paper.

C. Graphs

Pilot data whenever possible. If the graph is appropriate to the text, it should be submitted as a half-plate glossy photographic print, which means that all lines and points must be jet black on the original. Graphs are used essentially to bring out relationships among data, and should be reserved for that purpose. They are not ornaments. Graphs can provide profiles of data and trends which may not otherwise be understood easily in another form. Two curves of a graph may contain a total of 40 measurements which as a table would look pretty formidable; as a table the point might be lost anyway. There are certain rules to be observed:

1. Do not crowd everything into a single graph. Either have more than one graph or omit the less important facts (Fig. 21). Usually 3–4 lines on a graph are near the limit of intelligibility.

2. Remember that the size of any lettering on the original will have to be calculated for the reduction which occurs in the photographic print. Some journals prefer authors to inscribe letters on a sheet of clear cellophane placed over the print: the journal then uses the correct type which conforms to its own lithographic style. Therefore consult the editor's notes in the journal of choice at an early stage.

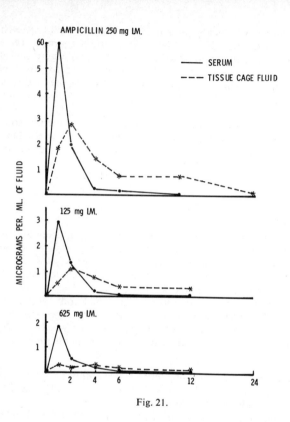

Fig. 21.

3. A decision often has to be made whether to join individual plots by straight or curved lines (Fig. 22). Curves look better but unless there are sufficient points to support them they may be grossly misleading. In Medicine, angular graphs are preferred for this reason,

and moreover, unjustified extrapolations should never be drawn in the finished illustration.

4. If the plots do not pass through the zero mark, then a broken line should be used to indicate this.

5. The abscissa and ordinate lines should always be calibrated.

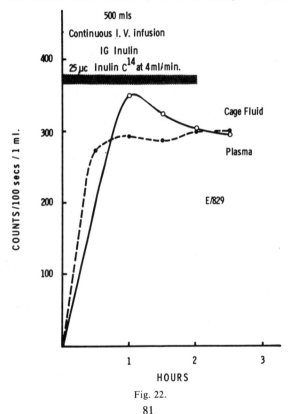

Fig. 22.

One should avoid the use of large numbers in any scale, such as 1000, 2000 but indicate them as 1, 2, etc., $\times 10^2$. The independent variables should be plotted on the horizontal axis and the dependent variable on the vertical axis. By convention, time is always on the horizontal axis.

6. If the graph becomes lop-sided, it may be worth substituting a logarithmic scale on one axis, but this must be clearly shown.

7. The usual symbols for plotting are $\times$, $\bigcirc$, $\square$, $\triangle$.

The last three can also be used as solid figures. If there is more than one graph in the paper, the same symbol must be used throughout for the same substance.

8. When asking yourself, 'Is this graph really necessary?', we suggest that it should always be retained if it relates to a new compound, if the results are open to several interpretations, and if the shape or peaks can be analysed mathematically.

D. Histograms

A bar chart may carry more impact than a graph. It is important to include the standard deviation or the standard error of the mean for each block, but it must be clear which statistic is being used. These are commonly provided as vertical lines centred on the horizontal line of the mean, but there is often no need to include the lower part of this line; a cleaner looking histogram will result. The figure for the number of observations should be included within the block unless they are all equal, in which case it should appear in the title. Although histograms commonly report a series of observations, this form of presentation can effectively record measurements on a single patient to disclose a pattern or shape which otherwise would not be evident. The disability of one finger in a patient with rheumatoid arthritis is shown in jet black in Figure 23. The table of absolute numbers is less attractive and less informative.

E. Photographs

Photographs may provide visual evidence of information better than any other form of illustration. Truth is not only stranger than

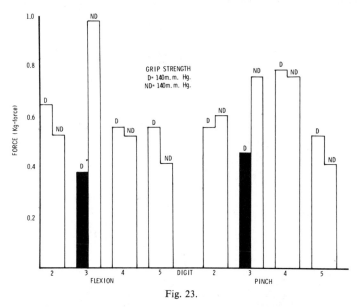

Fig. 23.

fiction, it is more telling. To see that a thing actually happened gives poignancy which mere description does not. Photographs are valuable for surface objects or procedures, but often disappointing elsewhere. They should be submitted as:

1. Half-plate prints on contrast and glossy paper.
2. The background should be plain, either white or black, and without distractions.
3. Skilful illumination should be used to provide shadows to impart a three dimensional quality.
4. Close-up pictures are generally more informative than panoramic views.
5. They should be unmounted and on the reverse in soft pencil

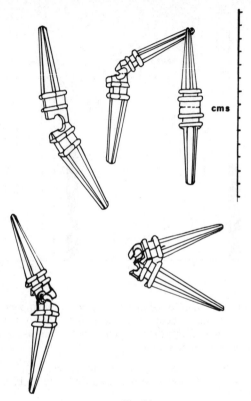

Fig. 24.

(2B) or felt pen should be marked for the printer, the 'top' to indicate the correct way up, and a figure number to correspond with that in the text. Never use a ball-point pen as it breaks the glaze and may spoil the block.

6. If several photographs are submitted it is economical to arrange them in groups for publication.

7. Remember that electron micrographs do not reproduce well, and for light microscopy a black and white print from a colour slide just will not do. In both, definitive areas should be indicated by arrows which are added to the prints later (Lettraset markers). Colour photographs, as prints and not submitted as transparencies, are very expensive to publish. Commonly the author is charged for their reproduction, so it is wise to negotiate the likely cost if they are essential for the publication. Finally, sometimes simple diagrams will disclose more than a photograph (Fig. 24).

F. Legends

Every photograph, diagram, histogram, and graph will require a legend, but tables only need an informative title. They should be typed on a separate sheet beginning with the number of the illustration: it is wasteful to use a separate sheet for each legend. If a description is supplied for each title it should be complementary to the text, not repetitive. Any wordy description should be put in the text. In the legend it may distract the reader too long from the main treatise and he will then have to go back to pick up the theme of the text after an unnecessary diversion. For illustrations of microscopy it is usual to give the stains used and the magnification, such as 'H and E × 40'; this abbreviation of haematoxylin and eosin at 40 magnifications is accepted generally. However, less well-known stains should be written in full. Legends are expensive to print and so should be kept brief; they should always be referred to in the text. A picture or a graph which is self-explanatory needs no caption. In this case, the list of illustrations should indicate 'Figure X—no legend'.

4. The Introduction

The introduction should be short and savoury so that the reader can get to the main body of the paper. It should be entertaining, easy reading, and give sufficient information to whet the appetite. It introduces the subject but does not develop it.

The introduction has 6 functions:

1. to make clear the subject of the paper, and to stress its importance;
2. to state the problem and clearly define the limits of the subject. (It is sometimes worth stating what you are *not* going to do.)
3. to give reasons for investigating this particular subject;
4. to set out the scope and general method of investigation, or to provide a quick review of the organization which follows;
5. to record the most significant finding so that the reader is alerted early and can assess the evidence for it as he reads;
6. to refer to the pertinent literature only so far as this bears on the introduction. Long historical reviews are dull and multiple references, which are more appropriate to the discussion, should not be included here.

Every literary man knows Bacon's essay which begins—'What is truth?', said jesting Pilate, and did not wait for reply'—an opening which is still fresh 300 years later. Dickens' first statement in 'A Christmas Carol'—'Marley was dead; to begin with'—produces by sheer incongruity a similar impact.

The importance of the opening statement of the introduction can hardly be over-emphasized. How can it be done successfully? There is no simple answer. In many ways it is the most important part of the paper, and is often the last to be rewritten. The beginning of the introduction should be employed to make the reader interested enough to read the whole work, and may set the tone and quality of the entire paper. It may vary in length from a single sentence to several pages. There are 7 possible ways to start the paper and we give an example for each:

1. Announce the subject immediately in the first paragraph. This is common in academic papers but usually too stiff and formal for many of us.

'Methods for the prevention of deep vein thrombosis have been slow to develop. On the assumption that stasis of blood is a major aetiological factor we designed a controlled clinical trial to investigate the use of intermittent compression of the legs during and after surgery.'

2. Use an opening statement which arouses the curiosity, surprise, or attention of the reader.

'Every year 10 people die unnecessarily at our hospital. They have had successful surgical operations and are looking forward to going home. Suddenly they are dead.'

3. Start by asking an important question, or even a series of questions which the paper will answer. The practice of completion 'by return' is a pleasing method which imparts symmetry and form to the finished article. The question may, of course, be rhetorical, and no answer be given.

'Why does silent thrombosis occur so often after surgical operations? How many people have undiagnozed but minor pulmonary emboli? We just do not know.'

4. Report a personal experience of a story which has detail relevant to the topic of the paper. Anecdotes and allusions are highly effective but in practice are difficult to write well.

'A young and promising architect had a large mole removed from his chest wall and the defect covered by a skin graft. Healing was uneventful, but some swelling of his left leg delayed his discharge from hospital for several weeks. Ten years later he is almost completely incapacitated by a large oedematous and ulcerated leg which limits his mobility. What had happened?'

5. Historical:

'In 1856 Virchow concluded that there were three factors responsible for venous thrombosis—stasis of blood flow, hypercoagulability of blood, and vessel intimal damage. A century later, we know very little more.'

87

6. State an informative fact which may be of importance to the welfare of the reader.

'Anyone over the age of 60 who undertakes a long journey by air is advised to spend some of the time moving about. The risk of thrombosis in the legs is very real, and may be fatal.'

7. Make a significant quotation from the literature, or a statement made by some other person. If you can puzzle your reader he is probably captured.

On a new technique for isotope scanning:

'The pancreas lies deeply in the abdomen. It cannot be seen, it cannot be felt, and it cannot be heard. How then is one to diagnose disease of this organ?'

Ambrose Paré, in despair of his ignorance, wrote: 'I dressed the wounds, God cured the patients.'

8. Give an outline précis of the paper. The summary can give a detailed synopsis if the journal normally places this at the end; if the summary is put at the beginning, such an introduction is repetitious.

9. A commonplace remark.

One of Belloc's essays began with 'I have a wealthy friend'. So one might start: 'My father died from thrombosis. He was only 49'.

There are several other ways of beginning and every author should think out the most appropriate to his subject. For inspiration, read the headlines on the front page of any daily newspaper: the editor has learned by experience how to capture the interest of his readers. If he does his job well, sales increase; if badly done, sales decline It's as simple as that.

5. The Main Data and Results

The reader is entitled to have the data presented in a logical order, which may not have been the order in which the work was done. We presume that the exercise was carried through to support or to state a new hypothesis.

There are 5 requisites for a useful (as opposed to useless) hypothesis, for it should:

1. explain the known facts;
2. be consistent with all the known facts;
3. be no more complex than necessary;
4. aid prediction of new facts and relationships;
5. be susceptible of verification or refutation.

The results may be presented as graphs, tables, and simple description. In science the object is precise measurement. Galileo said: 'measure what is measurable and make measurable what is not.' In the biological sciences we know that all measurements are inexact and the only way to describe this variability is to use statistics intelligently. The standard deviation is more elegant and more descriptive than the range; the mean is a better term than the average, and the standard error of the mean allows one to compare two or more sets of measurements with a real chance of obtaining the truth. Hence tests of significance which must be specified in tables or in the text (the 't' test, Chi-square, and other tests) become an integral part of recorded results. Statistical significance is not the same as importance. Statistics permit you to present all the data more simply and allow the reader to draw his own conclusions, which may not be the same as the author's. We also advise giving the number of observations in brackets when data are written in the script, so that the reader can understand the relevance of the information. For instance, 'serum proteins were 6.7 ± 1.7 G/100 ml (20) compared with 2.5 ± 1.2 G/100 ml (18) in tissue cages'. The fact that the difference between the protein concentrations is statistically highly significant ($P < 0.001$) can be interpreted as important because of the number of observations.

6. The Discussion

The section of the paper headed 'discussion' should conform to two rules:

(a) It should be no longer than is necessary to explain the implications of the work.

(b) It should be in three parts which are linked subtly so that it appears to be a short essay.

1. Interpretation

How can you explain what you have done, and what are the results? From this part will stem the main conclusions which must be based on evidence. Immaterial evidence should be omitted in the discussion but you can use supporting evidence from published work, and circumstancial evidence, such as observation made at the time the work was being done. It is important to be factual. Reference can and should be made to tables and graphs in the paper. Any qualifications of the conclusions and their importance should be clearly stated. A collection of facts is only of value when they either fit into a current hypothesis or support a new one: there is no purpose in discovering them otherwise.

2. Disputation

How does your work fit into the general body of knowledge of the subject? This is where references to published work will come. The claims of others can be argued and unsettled points disclosed.

3. Disquisition

What are the implications of your work for other disciplines, and how might they affect current practices? This is the section for opinions, philosophy, and a little theory, some of which may alert another man to plan further experiments or to propose a new hypothesis.

Although they may be written separately there should be a smooth flow from one facet to another. The gifted writer will find this section the most stimulating. It is not easy to do well, and should be examined most closely before the manuscript is typed. It should be a debate with yourself.

The Rules of Evidence

Before making conclusions it is advisable to examine the data and the discussion carefully, and to apply the rules of evidence. These differ little from the rules of civil law.

1. All the facts of the investigation should be disclosed. This does not mean that all detail of experiments must be included, but it is important to include abnormal results if these are not due to faults of technique.

2. The burden of proof and counter-proof lies with the author. While there is no such thing as absolute proof in science, the degree of proof needed varies with the type of work done.

3. There should be proof beyond reasonable doubt on the balance of probability, which means using statistics intelligently to support the original hypothesis.

4. Circumstancial evidence can be admitted provided that it is supported by documentary evidence from other publications.

5. Hearsay evidence is prohibited. Surmise, intuition, and guess-work, may be written in the discussion, along with personal opinions, but have no place in any conclusions.

6. In interpreting the results which appear to support your hypo-thesis, arguments for and against should both be adequately presented. Although you may think that the data presented are conclusive, another may argue otherwise, and set up experiments designed specifically to contradict your own conclusions.

When a judge sums up a case he recapitulates the facts that have been put before the jury and comments on the speeches of counsel (Fig. 25). He does not offer new evidence, but he does discuss both arguments, for the prosecution and for the defence. So too with scientific discussion.

Some Common Errors in Conclusions

To one man the conclusions from a piece of investigation are obvious, to another they are not. Errors are commonly made by mistaking parallelism for cause and effect, by missing the point, or

91

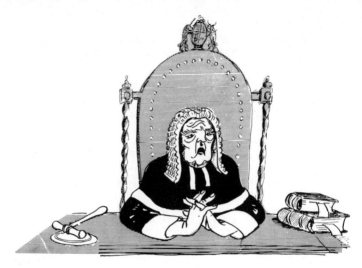

Fig. 25.

by begging the question. Too broad generalization may be drawn from too few facts. Because of prejudice the conclusions may be unwelcome, and therefore rejected.

7. Concluding the Paper

Hilaire Belloc commented that 'to begin at the beginning is, next to ending at the end, the whole art of writing'. How a writer begins will determine whether his reader bothers to go on; how he ends will determine whether the reader is satisfied or unconvinced. Anyone can stop writing but only a writer can finish.

There are 5 ways in which the author can bring his writing to a close:

1. End with a list of the main conclusions.

However slight the written contribution may be, most papers

should state one or more conclusions. There are 3 possibilities:

(a) The conclusions agree with what everyone already knows, and in this manner support contempory knowledge. This is the commonest finding, but no less worthy for that.

(b) The conclusions sustain ideas and views suspected to be true, but for which there was previously little corroborative evidence. Reputations are built this way.

(c) The findings are entirely new and have not been thought of before. Fortunate indeed is the author whose work comes into this category. The common response is disbelief, so that a further publication in defence of the new concept becomes imperative. Guyton's (1963) evidence that tissue fluid pressure is normally subatmospheric is a good example. By direct experimentation he refuted theoretical calculations which had been accepted by physiologists for nearly a century. Further publications from 1967 to 1972 became necessary, even though the essential facts received confirmation by others (Calnan et al., 1972 a. and b.)

2. Summarize what has been done and give the main findings. If the journal prints an abstract with the paper, any separate summary is unnecessary.

3. Use signal words such as 'finally', 'in conclusion', and 'lastly'.

4. Return to the beginning by answering the question in the opening statement of the introduction. Completion by return is an elegant way of closing. It follows a principle in art that form is everything.

5. Indicate what further work will be required to elucidate the problems which your work has uncovered.

8. The Summary

The wise man will make a short summary of every paper that he writes. It is an excellent discipline for it sharpens critical ability and teaches economy of words. A short clear summary not only makes reading easier, it also facilitates translation into foreign languages.

93

Many journals demand a summary, to be used either for the convenience of abstracting services or for the convenience of the reader. If the summary is placed at the beginning of the paper it is commonly called an 'abstract'. It should précis the content of the paper in 150–200 words, be interesting and meaty, and will include some of the conclusions. The exact number of words depends on the current practice of the journal. An abstract will thus influence the style of the introduction to the main paper. Its composition requires considerable skill and should indicate what was done, why it was done, how it was done, and the results—with simplicity and clarity. We condemn strongly the summary which says nothing: '100 cases were analysed, conclusions made and their importance discussed, etc.'

If the summary is normally placed at the end, almost as a completely separate offering, it should still be short and documentary. There is, however, some justification for enumerating the main conclusions because so many people tend to scan the title and then turn to the end of the paper before starting to read the article. To be greeted by say, three short and definitive conclusions encourages one to read on.

9. Acknowledgements

One would have thought it easy to say thank you when someone has done you a service, yet most people find it a difficult thing to say. Who should be thanked?

Throughout this book we have tried to emphasize the importance of consulting an experienced author for help. Ask your chief, if he has written several successful papers: do not consult him if he has not. If he helps by correcting the script and has materially aided its final form, this should be recognized in print. To curry favour by acknowledging a senior when he has done little is unworthy, for flattery corrupts both receiver and giver.

Technical help in experimentation should always be recognized and any financial help from a grant-giving body. The artist and the photographer generally do not sign their own work and it is the duty of the author to give them recognition.

The acknowledgements are usually placed at the end of the paper. A simple statement is all that is required; it should be short and factual, not long and flowery.

5

WRITING THE MANUSCRIPT

'Tolerance is only another name for indifference'—
Somerset Maugham

A man who is intelligent enough to be a surgeon is also intelligent enough to learn to write down what he wants to say in simple accurate terms (Macphail, 1911). Yet a surgeon is incapable of carrying out his job without the proper equipment. So too the author, and we suggest that his essential tools are:

1. A good dictionary. The 'Concise Oxford Dictionary' is small and manageable, but for more precise definitions the larger 'Shorter Oxford English Dictionary' in two volumes, is preferred.
2. Roget's 'Thesaurus of English Words and Phrases' is an invaluable source for alternative words, which may not necessarily carry the same connotations.
3. A book on English usage: Fowler is usually recommended but we like the small publication by Thomson and Irvine (1960).
4. A pad of plain paper of a quality that allows easy writing. A pen and not a pencil should be used if you value the time of your typist. We prefer a good ball-point pen with black ink.

We have no intention in this chapter of writing an English grammar. In our view grammar is of little importance, based as it is largely on rules of dead languages, when compared with clarity of meaning. The meaning of words varies with the context and the times in which we live for our language like our science is changing all the time. Yet to some people the normal rules of grammar have become more important than the need for clarity. Nicities of expression may not communicate the essential ideas that we wish to present, for there is a fundamental inexactitude of words as a means of communication.

96

For all that, grammar has its place: respect, not reverence, should be our attitude.

Many people appear to be incompetent to record an experiment in language, yet are well qualified in practice. The two common faults in such communication concern syntactical structure and semantics. The usual order in a sentence is noun, verb and object, but this may not be the most effective one. Word order can be rearranged but grammatical difficulties arise when qualifying phrases and subordinate clauses are introduced. For this reason alone there is probably more bad writing in medical journals than in any other kind of periodical. Bad writing is a slovenly habit.

Well-written papers do not just happen, they have to be worked for and it is only by writing often and critically that you will attain a higher standard. It is quite clear to us that doctors and civil servants as a class, both find the greatest difficulty in writing clearly and intelligently in the mother tongue. More than 20 years ago, Sir Ernest Gowers attempted to help the latter group in his book 'The complete plain words'. This little book is compulsory reading for all medical authors. What effect has it had on civil servants? We suspect very little for here is a quotation from the minutes of a local authority meeting in 1972:

'During a general discussion doubts were expressed about the possible revision of the valuation if contracts for purchase were not signed and exchanged within three months from the specific valuation, although the Clerk considered that in normal circumstances it should be possible for a contract to be signed within three months and that this would allow for consideration by a purchaser of his mortgage requirements, prior to signing a contract.'

Phew! Seventy words which may well have been said at the meeting, but surely need not be recorded thus. Although it is possible to parse this sentence and find the noun, verb and object, it does not make easy reading.

To write well it is necessary to acquire a wide and accurate vocabulary. This can only be accomplished by wide and constant reading, not only in medicine but also from newspaper editorials and good literature. Richard Asher (1972), was a skilful medical author who wrote with simplicity and precision on unusual clinical conditions, and the various works of Medawar (1969, 1970) should also be consulted. Unfamiliar words when they are seen should be looked up in the dictionary (Fig. 26) and it is good to acquire the regular habit of browsing through the dictionary: it can be opened at random if it is always on your desk. In this way it will become easy to learn the meaning and usage of effective and precise words, but one should avoid long words when a short one will do just as well.

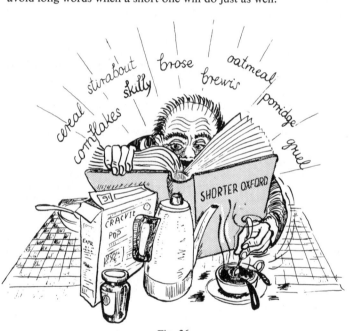

Fig. 26.

To become a painter you need more than a velvet beret and long hair; you have to learn how to see. This is not just a matter of talent, for it can be learnt if only there is a spark of enthusiasm: so too with writing.

The art of communication lies not only in presenting to the reader words that he can readily understand, but also the number he can assimilate in a reasonable time. The tally of publications which have been misinterpreted because they were too long and written in misguided language, is legion. We have tried to show that good writing requires careful planning, and follows the orderly sequence of accumulation, rumination, and execution. If you have followed our instructions so far, you will now be anxious to start writing.

1. The First Draft

Try to write the first draft in one sitting. You achieve unity this way. The danger in writing sections separately is that an uneven, jerky style will be produced. There is no need to worry about the quality of the English at this stage; competent workmanship, not art but craft, is required. Elegance and beauty of prose come later (Barzum, 1971). The object is to tell a simple tale well.

Do not repeat in tedious prose what is clear from tables and graphs. The data will speak for themselves, and you only have to point out the salient features. In the discussion leave out non-essentials, but discuss controversial issues lucidly and fairly.

When the first draft has been written, the list of references, tables, illustrations and their legends, should be clipped to the manuscript. Now you have a completed piece of work. The next job is to revise, correct and polish.

2. The First Revision: Revising the form

Put away the first draft for a week or two. It will need a lot of rewriting which is best done when it can be approached as though it were someone else's work. Ask yourself, 'How can I improve it? Is it concise? Is it clear?'

Read the manuscript through twice. The first time to find if it makes sense to you, the second to be critical. There are 4 aspects to look at:

(a) Alteration of structure.

Are major alterations necessary? If so, they should be written on separate sheets and the script cut and pasted accordingly. The object is to carry out a ruthless dissection of one's own work, viewing everything according to scientific principles. Familiarity with a subject can lead to glaring omissions, so ask yourself, 'Has anything important been left out?'

(b) Accuracy.

A writer's first paper may make or mar his reputation, so pay particular attention to the accuracy of the factual data reported. Accuracy is a matter of life and death in technical writing; without it nothing else matters. Your creditability as a serious writer can be destroyed by the incapacity to take pains, and by downright laziness. We have noticed that the same care in executing scientific experiments is not always matched in reporting. Common faults to watch are:

1. The misappropriation of quotations from published papers, by taking them out of context.

2. The misuse of words, technical or otherwise.

3. The misuse of statistics, either through ignorance or by an attempt to cheat (Huff, 1958).

4. Poor observations, frequently because important parts of the work were delegated to others who were incompetent to make them.

5. Making firm conclusions from inferences and 'value-judgements', a term which Mares (1967) reserves for 'informed opinion'. Conclusions must be clear and factual, verifiable statements.

(c) Order of presentation.

Re-examine the order in which you have presented the facts. If a paragraph should come earlier or later, cut it out with scissors and paste it to the new site. Clarity of purpose is the key to coherence; unity of thought makes for good reading.

(d) Examine the tables.

If necessary, combine or simplify them for clarity. Is the purpose of the table crystal clear? Is it informative? If not, leave it out and describe the results in the text.

If this is all to your liking, the next step is to revise the language.

In revising the language, six aspects of the manuscript should be looked at in detail.

3. Punctuation and Paragraphs

In writing, punctuation is necessary for comprehension. Thus, the full stop or period indicates the end of a sentence. The comma separates a word, phrase, or clause and so simplifies the meaning. The semicolon breaks up a longer sentence into smaller sentences which may be linked by the similarity of the subject matter. The colon provides a shorter break in a sentence and is often used to produce emphasis.

A common error is to omit the comma before a non-defining relative clause, which results in ambiguity for the reader so that he has to go back and re-evaluate the sentence. By contrast, the indiscriminate use of commas, particularly in long sentences, may puzzle the reader who now has to define for himself the qualifying clauses. The current trend is to reduce punctuation to a minimum, and this implies that sentences should be short and their meaning unequivocal.

The paragraph is the unit of thought in a group of sentences. When changing from one idea to another, a new paragraph should be started. Paragraphs also help to break up the printed page and so make reading easier. Single sentences however, should not form a paragraph unless conversation is being recorded. Emphasis is produced by the choice of words, not by isolating one sentence from its fellow, as in some modern novels.

4. Clarity

Clearness, conciseness and exactness, all contribute to clarity but they are somewhat vague terms and can be interpreted differently.

Clarity depends on:

1. A clear scheme.

Why did I do this work?
What did I find?
What does it mean?
Where does it lead?

The author who can answer these questions in simple unequivocal sentences has gone a long way to writing a readable clear paper. Articles often benefit from being written in the first person, they become more interesting, and if this is the most lucid way to record events there is no need to feel shy. But the great danger is pomposity in such prose. Clarity is acquired mainly by taking trouble and by writing to serve rather than to impress.

2. The choice of words—so try to use one instead of several, but do be sure that you know its exact and current meaning. True synonyms are rare, so avoid fancy words. Find the word which means exactly what you wish to say, which permits of only one interpretation —the correct one.

Here are some woolly nouns to avoid: area, character, conditions, field, levels, nature, problem, process, situation, structure, system, and some woolly verbs, achieved, attained, implemented, indicated, obtained, produced, required.

Vague qualifiers can usually be omitted to advantage: fairly, quite, rather, several, very, much. They deaden the style and clog the meaning.

Words used incorrectly as synonyms are:

amount   for concentration
content   for level
alternate   for alternative
minimal   for negligible
varying   for various

varied	for different
comprise	for constitute
distinctive	for distinct
effect	for affect

Words to avoid because they sound pompous and are commonly misused:

anticipate	better and simpler is expect
approximate	better and simpler is about
commence	better and simpler is begin
due to	better and simpler is owing to
demonstrate	better and simpler is show
extremities	better and simpler is hands/feet
hospitalize	better and simpler is admit to hospital
large number of	better and simpler is many
prior to	better and simpler is before
it may however be noted	better and simpler is nevertheless
it seems to the authors	better and simpler is we

3. Sentence construction.

Although we advise authors to write in a way that comes naturally, we wish to emphasize that one should avoid overstatement and a breezy manner; adding humour is generally dangerous—few can write this well. Simple constructions make for clarity, but a succession of short sentences give an unnatural staccato effect. The length of sentences should be varied but written in specific concrete language. It is often valuable to place the emphatic words at the end of the sentence, and to keep to the same active tense for the verbs. Poor writers employ phrases which tend to produce a succession of loose sentences; good authors employ effective words and cast aside the weak, worn and superfluous.

4. Thinking of the reader.

Will he understand what you wish to communicate? Have you written what you mean? If your paper has 6000 words, can you reduce it to 3000? An A4 sheet contains about 350 words in double spacing, a foolscap, about 400. What is superfluous? What is repetition? Brevity usually improves clarity.

5. Euphony. Does the paper read well? Does one idea flow from another in a logical order or will the reader find difficulty in following your argument? Would you describe your findings thus to a colleague? If not, then you have fallen into the trap of using unnatural and elaborate phrases. If you wish to correct this fault, we suggest that you read your paper to a tape-recorder and listen to the play-back. We advise that you wait at least one week before listening to your script, because the errors will be more obvious then.

5. Brevity

There are three rules for brevity:

1. It is your duty to the reader to be brief. Parsimony with words is never a vice and rarely a fault. The bulkiest publications are often short on facts and long on theory.

2. It is your duty to yourself to put the message over to the reader most economically. The important things in life require the simplest explanation. It is discourteous not to consider the time that the reader may require to read your prose, so avoid an orgy of the superfluous. Abbreviations should not be used unless a word or phrase is to be repeated several times. It is then permissible to record the abbreviation in brackets when the word or phrase is first written, and to use it from thence. This not only makes for economy of words but often facilitates quick reading.

3. Avoid phrases and try to substitute one word instead of many:

in order to—to
it is apparent that—hence
it is probable that—probably
a considerable amount of—much
a decreased number of—fewer
at some future time—later
are of the same opinion—agree

encountered more frequently—commoner
in a considerable number of cases—often.

For other instances, see Hawkins (1967) and current medical journals.

6. Interest

The reader's interest is maintained most readily by the author who has something worthwhile to report and writes it well. That extra sparkle to your paper can be added by:

1. Making each paragraph a coherent unit, and having a smooth transition from one paragraph to the next. In this way, successive paragraphs are linked together to produce continuous prose. Framing words such as first, second and third, often help to organize a paragraph.

2. Using short sentences after long ones, and it is important to vary the rhythm of writing to produce emphasis. A varied sentence style is apt to be more interesting. Sentence structure is determined largely by the manner in which you organize your ideas but it is often a good idea to place the important words you wish to emphasize at the end.

3. Using illustrations to most effect, if the picture will tell your reader more, and more vividly than words, what you wish to communicate to him. To this end illustrations may be numerous or few, detailed or sketchy.

4. Choosing words carefully with attention to their connotations for the reader.

5. Parellelism is among the most useful tools for a writer, but you must remember not to make conclusions of cause and effect from such examples. Antithesis is a neat way of handling contrasts.

6. Active verbs (and not the passive voice) improve the clarity and vigour of a sentence. Scholarly writing does not have to be impersonal, and the use of 'I' and 'we' can rapidly change the appeal of a sentence.

7. In providing definitions, give several concrete examples of the thing defined, and remember that fresh sharp images will help the reader to understand abstract relationships. Exposition explains, but judgement unfolds a question and measures the answer.

8. To be fully effective an argument must be not only well-reasoned but well-expressed. Argument and judgement are often very close, for rarely are all the facts on one side. No logical argument is better than the premises on which it rests, and the writer must define his meaning of important key words as soon as he introduces them.

9. Cut out the clichés. Here are some to avoid, a list to which you can add your own:

'There are several problems . . .
In the broadest possible terms . . .
meaningful relationships . . .
furthering the cause of good surgical practice in the general context of . . .
unable to accept the hypothesis in its present form . . .
On the surface this looks attractive, but in probing deeper . . .'

There are also a host of words which have lost their impact and are best avoided unless they are used correctly:—'overall, maximal, balanced, integrated, compatible, synchronized, calculated, functional, management, contingency, capability'—and many more current in medical and surgical journals. They strangle clear writing. Dean (1966) has a collection which he calls 'vogue words'.

7. Jargon

What is jargon? The Concise Oxford Dictionary defines jargon as 'unintelligible words, barbarous or debased language'. When one is told to avoid jargon in writing, commonly the advice is to avoid a mode of speech full of unfamiliar terms. This is the nub. To a doctor, a technical report in engineering appears to be full of jargon; the reverse is also true. We have therefore to distinguish between 'gibberish' and a 'technical vocabulary'. Elder (1954) argued that if the technical vocabulary of a science is jargon then all such authors must be condemned, for in no other way can they achieve clarity and conciseness of expression in writing. But what is the use of fine research if the results cannot be communicated to all who might benefit? Publication is the end product of research, for without it research becomes sterile.

In medicine, technical terms have been defined and are recorded in special dictionaries. These words have been constructed and designed to serve the writer's needs with precision and economy. Some words, of course, have different shades of meaning, and when used in statements their precise meaning should be explained. This implies that simple words should be substituted for the technical term where possible; they should, as a courtesy to the reader, for the object is not to produce an orgy of difficult words for economy, but to write clearly.

The misuse of scientific terms, the attempt to impress, the deliberate invention of a new word, and the promotion of long words instead of simple everyday terms—these all constitute bad jargon, a lazy habit. We must agree with McAllister (1955) that technical terms with precise meanings are desirable for communication between experts, provided the audience understands them. He calls this 'accepted scientific jargon'; we prefer 'technical terms' and have tried to separate the good from the bad.

Pei (1970) advised that a word which had become debased should be treated like counterfeit money—'Don't accept it, and don't pass it on'. We entirely agree. To our mind, jargon is as much the padding, the obscurity and the roundabout way of describing what you want to say, as the misuse of scientific terms: and it is noticeable that a surfeit of such jargon disfigures so many official documents—the very papers which above all should be crystal clear.

8. Rules for Numbers

1. Do not use numerals at the beginning of a sentence.

2. Do not use two numerals in juxtaposition: it is better to write 20 four inch test tubes', and not '20 4 inch . . .'.

3. Do not use numerals when referring to approximations—about one hundred patients.

4. Use words for numbers below ten, and numerals for larger numbers, and for all figures, diagrams and tables, unless the journal gives specific instructions otherwise.

5. Observe the correct abbreviations for units of measurement (see Ellis, 1971: Jaggi, 1969).

6. Use Arabic and not Roman numerals unless the journal specifies their use, commonly for tables.

9. Having it Typed

If you have followed our advice so far, your manuscript will not be a pretty thing. Sheets will be gummed together, corrections and additions will be evident. Yet it will be readable, correct and in order. Now is the time to re-number the pages, and add a covering note for the guidance of your typist, for all manuscripts must be typed:

1. Have *everything* double-spaced.

2. Leave ample margins all round: 3–4 cm is not excessive for the text.

3. Use good quality paper for the top copy.

4. Have at least three copies typed; you will need one for your files anyway. If there are several authors, each is entitled to a copy of the typescript and tables.

5. Tables, legends and references must all be typed on separate sheets. Each table requires one sheet and must carry a number and title. Do not crowd tables.

When all is done, read through the typescript of the first carbon copy word by word. Correct errors in coloured ink. If there are many corrections on one page, say more than six, it is considerate to the editor to have this page retyped. If at this stage some parts are not to your satisfaction, rewrite them. If you are considerate you will alter sentences so that only one page needs to be retyped and not the whole paper.

Finally, ask a friend to read it through. The object is not to produce great literature but to write so that your meaning is clear to other doctors who may not practice in your field of work, and to those whose language is not English.

6

THE 10 COMMANDMENTS

1. Arrange the material.
2. Have a clear intention.
3. Think before you write.
4. Write with purpose and accuracy.
5. Revise, revise, revise.
6. Improve the order.
7. Improve the English.
8. Don't imitate.
9. Publish when satisfied.
10. Do better next time.

REFERENCES AND FURTHER READING

FURTHER READING, REFERENCES TO PAPERS

Alexander, R. S. (1953). 'Trends in Authorship', *Circulation Res.*, **1,** 281–283.

Allen, E. M. (1960). 'Why are Research Grant Applications Disapproved?' *Science*, **132,** 1532–1534.

Asher, R. (1951). 'Manchausen Syndrome', *Lancet*, **1,** 339–341.

Asher, R. (1958). 'A Woman with the Stiff-man Syndrome', *Brit. Med. J.*, **1,** 265–266.

Asher, R. (1959). 'Making sense', *Lancet*, **2,** 259–265.

Baker, J. R. (1955). 'Style in Scientific Papers', *Nature (Lond.)*, **176,** 851–852.

Barber, A. S., Barraclough, E. D. and Gray, W. A. (1972). 'Closing the Gap Between the Medical Reasearcher and the Literature (on Medlars)', *Brit. Med. J.*, **1,** 368–370.

Barzum, J. (1971). 'So Long as Doctors have to Think', *Bull. N.Y. Acad. Med.*, **47,** 229–235.

Dean, R. L (1966) 'Dr Wilders Catalogue of Vogue Words', *J. Amer. Med. Assn.*, **196,** 70–71.

Elder, J. D. (1954). 'Jargon—good and bad', *Science*, **119,** 536–538.

Jaggi, W. (1969). 'The Manuscript', 6th Edn., Karger, Basel. (A guide for authors preparing manuscripts for Karger publications. Gives a list of abbreviations for the names of journals, units of measurement, and good advice on illustrations. The notes on presentation do not apply to all journals but are worth noting.)

McAllister, D. T. (1955). 'Is There Accepted Scientific Jargon?', *Science*, **121,** 530–532.

Macphail A. (1911). 'Style in Medical Writing', *Canad. Med. Assoc. J.*, **1,** 70–73.

Merrith, D. H. (1963). 'Grantmanship: An Exercise in Lucid Presentation', *Clin. Res.*, **11,** 375–377.

Roland C. G. (1971). 'Personal View', *Brit. Med. J.*, **2,** 301.

Thornton, J. L. (1971). 'Medical Libraries and Research', *Brit. J. Hosp. Med.*, Oct. 485–490.

Welbourn, R. B. (1966). 'The Training and Education of a Surgeon', *Proc. Roy. Soc. Med.*, **59**, 934–936.

Woodford, F. P. (1967). 'Sounder Thinking Through Clearer Writing', *Science*, 156, 743–745.

REFERENCES TO BOOKS

Asher, R. (1972). *Richard Asher Talking Sense*, Edited by F. Avery Jones, Pitman, London. (Enjoyable reading if only for the unusual subjects discussed, the subtle wit and breadth of knowledge. The scrupulous use of the English language and economy of words should appeal to the modern medical author.)

Baker, C. (1961). *A Guide to Technical Writing*, Pitman, London.

Beveridge, W. I. B. (1965). *The Art of Scientific Investigation*, Mercury, London. (Very readable and full of good sense.)

Calnan, J. and Barabas, A. (1973). *Speaking at Medical Meetings— A Practical Guide*, Heinemann, London. (A clear exposition of how to prepare and present a lecture. Recommended—naturally!)

Carey, G. V. (1971). *Mind the Stop*, Penguin, Harmondsworth. (All you need to know about punctuation in 124 pages.)

Cohen, J. M. and Cohen, M. J. (1969). *Penguin Dictionary of Modern Quotations*, Penguin, Harmondsworth. (Useful for composing the introduction.)

Cooper, B. M. (1964). *Writing Technical Reports*, Penguin, Harmondsworth. (Mainly for scientists and engineers, but good reading for all doctors.)

Ellis, G. (Editor) (1971). *Units Symbols and Abbreviations. A Guide for Biological and Medical Editors and Authors*, London, Royal Society of Medicine.

Gunning, R. (1968). *The Technique of Clear Writing*, Revised Edition, McGraw-Hill, New York. (Worth consulting for examples of his 'fog-index'.)

114

Huff, D. (1958). *How to Lie with Statistics*, Gollancz, London. (A humorous account of the many erroneous ways of using statistics; unfortunately still topical.)

Kane, T. S. and Peters, L. J. (1969). *Writing Prose*, 3rd Edn., Oxford University Press, New York. (An excellent analysis of the prose of various authors. Well worth reading.)

McNalty, A. (1965). *Butterworths Medical Dictionary*. (An essential reference for medical terms.)

Mares, C. (1966). *Communication*, English Universities Press, London. (A good account of how to communicate.)

Medawar, P. B. (1969). *The Art of the Soluble*, Penguin, Harmondsworth. (A collection of essays, finely written, on various aspects of biology.)

Miller, H. (1968). *B.M.A. Planning Unit: Research Funds Guide*, B.M.A. Publications, London. (A comprehensive guide to sources of finance for research in the U.K. and a note on applying for grants.)

Morton, L. T. (1964). *How to Use a Medical Library*, 4th Edn., Heinemann, London. (Essential reading for the serious medical writer.)

Palmer, F. (1971). *Grammar*, Penguin, Harmondsworth. (An adult view of English grammar.)

Pei, M. (1970). *Words in Sheep's Clothing*. (*How People Manipulate Opinion by Distorting Word Meanings*), Allen & Unwin, London. (A light-hearted account by a linguist. Mainly aimed at the U.S.A. but we are fast catching up. Science and pseudo-science in chapter nine. Entertaining reading.)

Quiller-Couch, A. (1958). The Oxford Book of English Prose, Clarendon Press, Oxford. (An anthology from earliest times. The works of well-known writers are quoted in 2–3 pages and so ideal for occasional reading.)

Roget's Thesaurus, Revised by R. A. Dutch (1968). Penguin, Harmondsworth. (Indispensable.)

Roueché, B. (1966). *Dossier of Medical Detection*, Gollancz, London. (Case reports written as detective stories. Creates a gripping narrative from simple clinical details. So why be dull?)

Strunk, W. (1959). *The Elements of Style*, Macmillan, London. (A readable and short account on how to acquire good style in writing.)

Thompson, R. D. and Irvine, A. H. (1960). *Everyday English Usage*, Collins, London. (Describes correct usage of words and figures of speech in 180 pages.)

Thorne, C. (1970). *Better Medical Writing*, Pitman, London. (Good sense.)

S. F. Trelease (1958). *How to Write Scientific and Technical Papers*, Williams & Wilkins, Baltimore. (Mainly for scientists but much applies to medicine.)

E. B. Wilson (1952). *An Introduction to Scientific Research*, McGraw-Hill, London.

F. P. Woodford (Editor) (1968). *Scientific Writing for Graduate Students. A Manual on the Teaching of Scientific Writing*, Rockefeller University Press, New York.

INDEX